Photodermatology

Edited by

James Ferguson MD, FRCP

Consultant Dermatologist
Photobiology Unit
Ninewells Hospital
Dundee, Scotland, UK

Jeffrey S Dover MD, FRCPC

Associate Clinical Professor of Dermatology
Yale University School of Medicine
and
Adjunct Professor of Medicine
Dartmouth Medical School
and
Director, SkinCare Physicians of Chestnut Hill
Massachusetts, USA

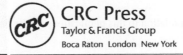

CRC Press
Taylor & Francis Group
Boca Raton London New York

CRC Press is an imprint of the
Taylor & Francis Group, an **informa** business

Acknowledgments

We are enormously grateful to the staff members of the Dundee Photobiology Unit, in particular to Maureen Hughes, Lynn Fullerton, Karen Stephen, and her staff. Many thanks also go to all the contributors who have given generously of their time to produce this book.

CRC Press
Taylor & Francis Group
6000 Broken Sound Parkway NW, Suite 300
Boca Raton, FL 33487-2742

© 2006, 2010 by Taylor & Francis Group, LLC
CRC Press is an imprint of Taylor & Francis Group, an Informa business

No claim to original U.S. Government works

ISBN-13: 9781840761351 (pbk)

Contents

Preface

Photodermatology, the study of the biological effects of ultraviolet and visible light on the skin, has, as an area of knowledge, expanded rapidly over the past 20 years.

Following introductory chapters on elementary photobiology and photophysics, equipment, and photoprotection, this book focuses on the clinical presentation, investigation, and discussion of treatment options for various photodermatoses (light-sensitive skin disorders), along with a discussion of the rapidly evolving subject of cutaneous laser surgery. Doctors and nurses have an important role to play not only in the diagnosis of the photodermatoses, but also in the administration of phototherapies. More recent additions under the umbrella of photodermatology include laser and photodynamic therapy.

This book provides an introduction into these various areas. It is intended to whet your appetite and to stimulate further interest in these areas. While this book is primarily photographic in content, a significant amount of standardized text has been included to provide an up-to-date view of what is a rapidly changing subject.

James Ferguson and Jeffrey S Dover

Contributors

Paula Beattie MRCP
Specialist Registrar, Ninewells Hospital, Dundee, UK

David Bilsland DCH, FRCP
Consultant Dermatologist, Southern General Hospital
Glasgow, UK

Alyson Bryden MRCP
Specialist Registrar, Ninewells Hospital, Dundee, UK

Colin Clark FRCP
Consultant Dermatologist, Glasgow Royal Infirmary
Glasgow, UK

Robert S Dawe MD, FRCP
Consultant Dermatologist, Ninewells Hospital, Dundee, UK

Jeffrey S Dover MD, FRCP
Associate Clinical Professor of Dermatology
Yale University School of Medicine, Director, SkinCare Physicians
of Chestnut Hill, Massachusetts, USA

James Ferguson MD, FRCP
Consultant Dermatologist, Photobiology Unit
Ninewells Hospital, Dundee, UK

Girish Gupta FRCP
Consultant Dermatologist, Monklands Hospital, Airdrie, UK

Sally Ibbotson MD, FRCP
Senior Lecturer in Dermatology/Consultant Dermatologist,
Ninewells Hospital, Dundee, UK

Graham Lowe FRCP
Consultant Dermatologist, Ninewells Hospital
Dundee, UK

Irene Man MRCP
Specialist Registrar, Ninewells Hospital
Dundee, UK

Harry Moseley PhD, FInstP
Consultant Photophysicist, Ninewells Hospital
Dundee, UK

Alexander J Stratigos MD
Assistant Professor of Dermatology/Venereology
National University of Athens Medical School
Athens, Greece

Nicholas J Wainwright MA (Oxon), FRCP
Consultant Dermatologist, Monklands Hospital
Airdrie, UK

Julie Woods BSc(Hons), PhD
Non-Clinical Lecturer, Ninewells Hospital
Dundee, UK

1 Introduction

James Ferguson

Photobiology is the study of the effects of non-ionizing radiation on living systems (1) and as such reflects all types of interaction of light with micro-organisms, plants and animals. Photomedicine is primarily concerned with diagnostic and therapeutic photobiology. This chapter is particularly related to introducing the clinical area of photodermatology, the study of the effects of non-ionizing radiation on predominantly the human skin.

There is a wide range of ultraviolet sources of which the most important is sunlight. Artificial light can be electric discharge, incandescent or fluorescent, with a wide variety of types present in the home and work environment. Our sun is one of many billions of similar stars. Electromagnetic irradiation emitted from the nuclear fusion reaction within the core takes nearly a million years to emerge at the sun's surface but then only 9 minutes to reach the earth.

On the basis of optical filters, ultraviolet has historically been subdivided into UVC, UVB and UVA wavelengths. In themselves, these bands do not indicate the limits of any biologic effect; they merely describe a numerical subdivision. In fact, within the literature there is a wide variety of waveband definitions and therefore it is always important to check which wavelength range is being used when you are reading a particular article. While in some ways it would be best if only

nanometers were described – for this is what optical physicists tend to use, so avoiding the artificial subdivisions of UVA, B and C – common usage dictates that the terminology will persist.

With a wide variety of biologic effects produced by different wavelengths, a population's susceptibility to a sunlight-sensitive skin disease will naturally vary (photodermatosis) according to a number of environmental factors. These include latitude, time of year, time of day, altitude, local pollution, and reflectant factors such as snow.

Sunlight is ultimately responsible for the majority of our energy and in particular is essential for growth of plants and therefore of vital importance in the food chain. Although in Genesis I *(The Holy Bible)*, it states that God said "Let there be light and there was light, and God saw that it was good", in fact sunlight has a range of positive and negative biologic effects *(Table 1.1)*.

It is hardly surprising therefore that, given its vital influence upon our lives, sun-worshipping cultures were common both close to the equator, such as Central America and North Africa, and even at latitudes away from the equator, such as the solar worship represented by the circle within the Celtic Cross (2), and reflect the recognition of the importance of light within these societies.

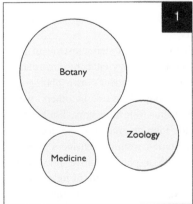

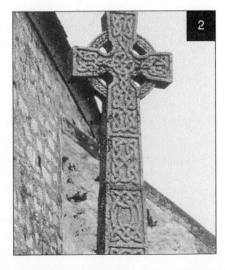

1: Photobiology: the study of non-ionizing radiation in living systems.
2: The Celtic Cross.

Table 1.1: Sunlight

Positive
- Photosynthesis
- Vision
- Vitamin D synthesis
- Killing pathogens
- Warmth
- Treatment of disease

Negative
- Biocidal action
- Sunburn
- Skin damage
- Carcinogenesis
- Photodermatoses
- Photosensitization
- Mutations

Within the chapters of this text, photodermatology is sub-divided into diagnostic and therapeutic aspects. Within the diagnostic group (3), a range of disease possibilities exist. With any referral center, the pattern as seen in *Table 1.2* and **4** will only approximately reflect the incidence; they are much more likely to reflect the need for investigation and the perceived need for investigation based on the severity of the affected patient.

Within the diagnostic range, a number of distinct groups exist. These include *idiopathic* which, although increasingly thought to have an immunologic basis, still in general needs to have evidence of the allergen and the type of the immune reaction defined. The genophotodermatoses are those genetically determined disorders; the porphyrias represent a mental/combination origin. Drug- and chemical-induced photosensitivity reactions are increasingly common as the number of therapeutic agents in use has increased. Photo-aggravation is commonly seen with a wide range of conditions when either patients report an exposed site problem or there is a clear history of summer seasonal activity, although they do not in general show true photosensitivity.

When you are considering each disease, it is useful to have in mind a simple schematic diagram (**4**). This allows release of information in terms of our current mechanistic understanding and identifies key facts that we need to know about each condition, even though many remain unknown at present. These include causal wavelengths, and the site and nature of the photon-absorbing chemical chromophore. The type of photochemistry that ensues gives details of the mediator release and subsequent inflammatory response reducing substrate damage with characteristic individual disease clinical features. This diagram is also of value in clarifying what can be done regarding therapy at each step in the pathogenesis.

Within the Dundee photodermatology clinic, history taking is an important exercise. With the photodermatoses a number of key questions can help tease out the role of sun and artificial light. It is important to define:
- the relationship to sunlight, whether it is direct or transmitted by window glass or clothing
- the minimum amount of light that can induce the problem
- the seasonal distribution, and
- the timing of onset and clearance.

Symptoms are often helpful in pointing towards specific diseases as is the patient's description of morphology. Careful history of drug/chemical exposure within the total home/recreation/work environments is often key to unraveling a difficult patient's diagnosis. Awareness of the fact that many patients do not regard some drugs as being worthy of mentioning should allow identification of such diagnoses as quinine photosensitivity.

The clinical presentation of the photodermatoses is of great distinguishing value. While morphology, either by direct clinical examination or by examining a patient's own photograph, can make the diagnosis straightforward. In others, where there is lack of clear information from the history, distribution of a photosensitive eruption may be crucial to the decision to put a patient through the time-consuming business of photo-investigation. Patients with a photosensitive presentation may show characteristic facial involvement of light-exposed areas and relative sparing of photoprotected sites, such as around eyes, below the nose and beneath the chin (**5–10** continued on to page 8). When you are examining back of neck and behind the ears, other sites of involvement and

Table 1.2: Dundee Photobiology unit: diagnoses 1971 – March 2004

Type	Numbers of diagnoses
Idiopathic	
Polymorphic light eruption	2022
Chronic actinic dermatitis	661
Actinic prurigo	120
Solar urticaria	104
Hydroa vacciniforme	30
Genophotodermatoses	
Xeroderma pigmentosum	12
Bloom syndrome	–
Cockayne syndrome	1
Rothmund Thomson disease	1
Harnup disease	–
Porphyrias	
Erythropoietic protoporphyria	50
Porphyria cutanea tarda	47
Other porphyrias	
Drug-induced photosensitivity/ phototoxicity	212
Photocontact dermatitis	109
Photo-aggravated dermatoses	744
Undiagnosed	412
Others	286
TOTAL DIAGNOSES	**4830**

sparing become clear. The scalp with sparing of a hair-bearing photoprotective area, coupled with involvement of the back of the hands and proximal phalanges of the fingers with sparing between the fingers and a cut-off at the clothing-protected wrist are important features to search for. Occasionally you might see striking photoprotection on areas protected by a watch or spectacle frame. In others, visible wavelength penetration of the white but not the dark pattern of clothing can be revealing.

Further reading

Frain-Bell W. *Cutaneous Photobiology*. Oxford University Press, 1985.

Hawk JLM. *Photodermatology*. Oxford University Press, 1999.

Magnus IA. *Dermatological Photobiology: Clinical and Experimental Aspects*. Blackwell Scientific Publications, 1976.

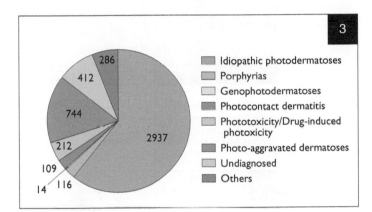

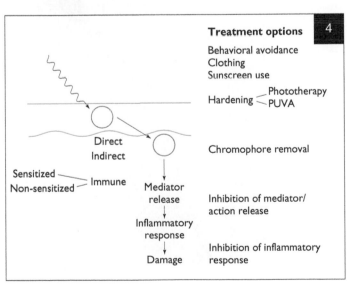

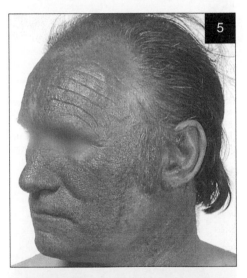

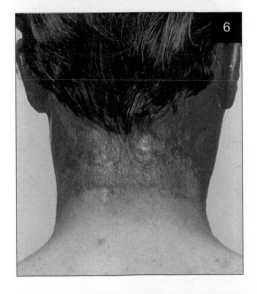

3: Photobiology unit idiopathic diagnoses.
4: Treatment options.
5: Exposed site dermatitis with sparing beneath sideburns, chin and side of neck.
6: Chronic actinic dermatitis showing collar and clothing protection.

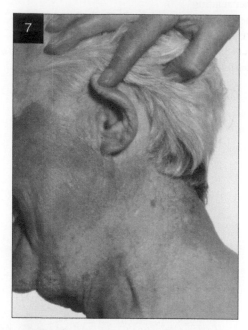

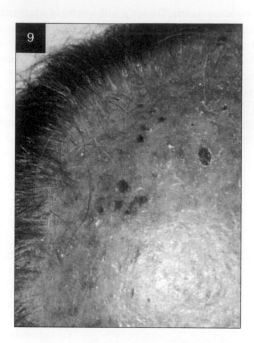

7: Notice the sparing of the shadow site behind the ear and cut-off at the neck in this chronic actinic dermatitis patient.

8: Back of hand involvement with relative sparing of the distal phalanges in a patient with thiazide photosensitivity.

9: Involvement of the bald area of scalp with sparing of the hair-bearing area in chronic actinic dermatitis.

10: Involvement of exposed as well as clothing-covered sites in chronic actinic dermatitis.

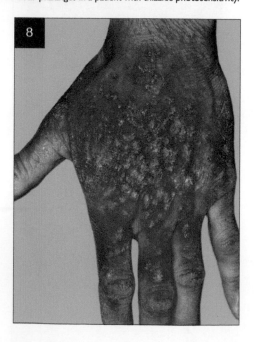

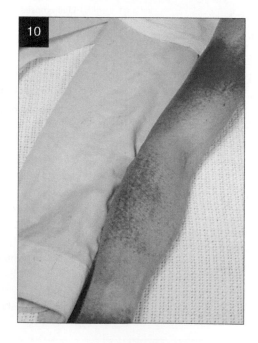

2 Elementary Photobiology and Photophysics

Harry Moseley

The spectrum

The electromagnetic (em) spectrum ranges from very short wavelength cosmic rays through X-rays, γ rays, ultraviolet (UV), visible, infrared to radiofrequency (RF) (11). The various types of em radiation differ with respect to their wavelength, which is simply the distance between the crests of the waveform (12). UV, visible and infrared radiation are collectively known as optical radiation. Light is, by definition, em radiation within the visible band.

Like any other transverse wave, there is a simple relation between wavelength (λ), velocity (c) and frequency (f):

$$\lambda = c/f$$

The UV region has been subdivided in several ways, the most common being that adopted by the International Commission on Illumination (Commission Internationale de l'Eclairage, CIE), which is:

UVA 315–400 nm
UVB 280–315 nm
UVC 100–280 nm.

Some authors take 320 nm as the boundary between UVA and UVB. UVA may be sub-divided into:

UVA1 340–400 nm
UVA2 315–340 nm.

Radiation of wavelength >200 nm is of little biologic significance because of its high absorption in air.

In 1901, Max Planck introduced the quantum theory and the concept that em radiation could be described as being emitted like discrete (quantized) packets of energy, called photons. He postulated that the energy (E) was proportional to the frequency. This has given rise to the wave/particle duality of light (12). Although they are fundamentally different ways of describing the same phenomenon, the photon and wavelength description may be related by the equation:

$$E = hf = hc/\lambda$$

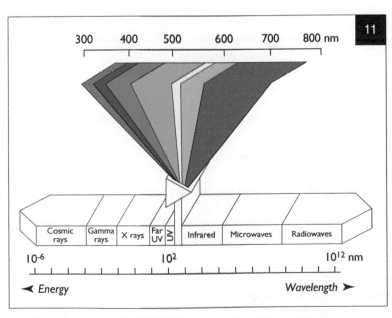

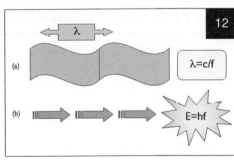

11: The electromagnetic spectrum. Wavelength and frequency are inversely related.

12: Light may be considered to act (a) like a wave characterized by wavelength, or (b) like a bullet called a photon with energy proportional to frequency. (See text for description of symbols.)

where h is Planck's constant (6 x 10³⁴ Joule seconds), c is the speed of light (2.998 x 10⁸ m/s in vacuum), f is frequency (Hz) and λ wavelength (m). Using this formula, the energy of a single photon corresponding to different wavelengths across the em spectrum may be determined. This is shown in **11**. Photon energy is expressed in units of electron volts (eV).

It is clear from this that a short wavelength photon carries more energy than that of a longer wavelength. For example, at a wavelength of 100 nm the corresponding photon energy is 12.4 eV, and at 400 nm it is 3.1 eV. UV through RF radiation is often regarded as non-ionizing radiation because the photon energy is considered to be insufficient to cause ionization. Although this is generally true, under certain conditions of high energy density, ionization may occur. Excimer lasers, for example, emit laser radiation in the UV region and are capable of causing ionization.

Radiometric quantities

In the UV part of the spectrum, optical radiation is measured using radiometric quantities, which are purely physical. Within the visible region, evaluation is described in photometric units, which incorporate the response of the human eye.

The unit of energy is the joule (J). Power is the rate at which energy is delivered and it is measured in watts (W). These two quantities are simply related:

$$\text{energy (J)} = \text{power (W)} \times \text{time (s)}$$

and, similarly:

$$W = J/s.$$

Dose is often expressed in terms of energy per unit area (J/m², mJ/cm², and so on). Irradiance (W/m², mW/cm², and so on) is the rate at which energy is delivered to unit area. As might be expected:

$$\text{dose (mJ/cm}^2) = \text{irradiance (mW/cm}^2) \times \text{time(s)}$$

If dose is prescribed in joules cm², to calculate the required exposure time, use the following equation:

$$\text{exposure time (s)} = \frac{\text{prescribed dose (J/cm}^2) \times 1000}{\text{irradiance (mW/cm}^2)}$$

Irradiance is sometimes referred to as intensity but this is incorrect as intensity is defined as power per unit solid angle. Also, other quantities such as fluence and fluence rate, although similarly expressed in J/m² and W/m² respectively, should not be employed, as they use the concept of additive backscatter.

The term spectral irradiance is the irradiance per unit wavelength (mW/cm²/nm). "Spectral" implies consideration of the wavelength dependency of the quantity. So, irradiance refers to exposure over a specified range of wavelengths, for example UVA or UVB irradiance; spectral irradiance is the irradiance per nanometer at a particular wavelength, for example as plotted in the spectral output from a lamp.

Some commonly used radiometric quantities and units are summarized in *Table 2.1*.

Table 2.1: Radiometric quantities and units

Quantity	Unit	Definition
Radiant energy	joule (J)	The total energy delivered by a radiation field
Radiant power/flux	watt (W)	The rate at which radiant energy is transferred from one region to another by the radiation field
Radiant exposure/dose	J/m²	Energy per unit area received by a surface
Irradiance	W/m²	The radiant power per unit area received by a surface
Spectral irradiance	W/m²/nm	The radiant power per unit area per unit bandwidth received by a surface
Fluence	J/m²	At a given point, the radiant energy incident on a small sphere divided by the cross-sectional area of that sphere
Fluence rate	W/m²	At a given point, the radiant power incident on a small sphere divided by the cross-sectional area of that sphere

Sunlight

There is a significant difference between the extraterrestrial spectrum and observations at sea level, the difference below 315 nm being of considerable biologic significance. Two-thirds of the energy from the sun outside the earth's atmosphere penetrates to ground level and only about 5% of this is UV radiation (**13**). The annual variation in extraterrestrial radiation is <10%, but the modifying effect of the earth's atmosphere is of greater significance (**14**). The stratospheric ozone layer absorbs wavelengths of <320 nm. It is essentially responsible for the lower cut-off wavelength of 290 nm at ground level and also absorbs 70–90% of UVB from the sun. Public concerns over ozone depletion became widespread following observations of the so-called ozone hole in Antarctica in the mid 1980s. This has sparked political initiatives, particularly the Montreal Protocol, aimed at eliminating the production and use of chlorofluorocarbons (CFCs) and other gases thought to be the principal cause of ozone depletion.

The UV levels from sunlight are strongly dependent on proximity to the equator, season of the year, and time of day since all of these factors contribute to the effective path length of sunlight through the absorbing layers of the earth's atmosphere. A meta-analysis of risk factors for cutaneous melanoma supported the intermittent exposure hypothesis: a positive association for intermittent sun exposure and an inverse association with a high continuous pattern of sun exposure.[4]

Absorption of radiation

The principle that radiation must be absorbed before a photochemical event can occur is fundamental to understanding photochemistry and photobiology and is known as the First Law of Photochemistry. Each molecule has a characteristic absorption spectrum, which can be considered as a plot of the probability that a photon will be absorbed against wavelength. The shape of the absorption spectrum of a molecule is determined by its particular electronic configuration plus environment. When a photon has been absorbed, there is an energy conversion and the molecule becomes electronically excited or, if the electron is removed, then photo-ionization takes place.

Excited electronic states

Electrons are negatively charged and spinning. When a molecule is in its ground state, electron spins are paired to give the ground electronic singlet state. If an electron is excited without change of spin, the electron is raised to an excited singlet state. If, in addition, it undergoes a change of spin, the resultant excited electronic state is termed a triplet state, so called because application of a magnetic field splits it into three levels. The terms "singlet" and "triplet" refer to what is called the "multiplicity" of the electronic state. All excited singlet states are associated with a triplet state, which is of lower energy. Most molecules are in the singlet state in their ground state, but oxygen, for example, is a ground state triplet molecule.

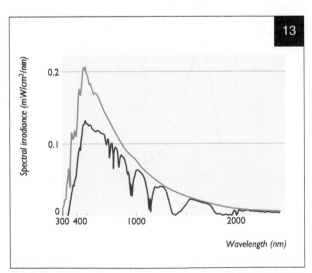

13: Spectral irradiance from the sun outside the earth's atmosphere and at sea level.

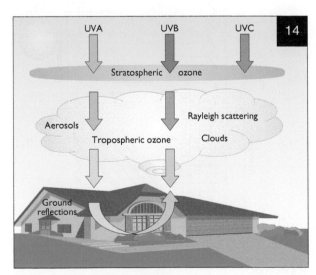

14: Variation of irradiance from sunlight.

On absorption of light, molecules are promoted from their singlet ground state to singlet excited states. Since electron energy levels are quantized, the energy (and hence wavelength) of the absorbed photon also can have discrete values only. The molecule also exhibits vibrational and rotational motions, which are likewise quantized. So, the total change of energy on absorption of a photon is the sum of the changes in the number of quanta of electronic, vibrational and rotational levels. Electronic quanta are larger than vibrational, which are larger than rotational. These states are shown in an energy level diagram, called a Jablonski diagram (15).

Fluorescence and phosphorescence

A molecule in an electronic excited state will lose energy and return to the ground state. One way of doing this is by way of internal conversion, which means that the molecule drops from a low vibrational level of an excited electronic state to a high vibrational level of the lower electronic state, and eventually loses its excess energy by collision. In this case energy is released as heat. Alternatively, it can emit a photon

in the form of fluorescence and return to the ground state. The fluorescence spectrum is shifted to longer wavelengths ("to the red") compared to the absorption spectrum. This is called Stokes' Law.

The excited singlet state is short-lived. On the other hand, the excited triplet state is more stable. So, another possible outcome is for the electron to undergo a change of spin (called intersystem crossing) and drop into the excited triplet state, from which it may decay by photon emission over a longer period of time to the ground state. Whereas typically fluorescence occurs in nanoseconds, the triplet lifetime may be as long as several seconds. The long-lived triplet emission is called phosphorescence. The phosphorescence spectrum lies at longer wavelengths than the fluorescence spectrum (16).

Photosensitization

When an absorption spectrum exhibits more than one peak, it indicates a corresponding number of excited states, which can be reached by irradiation of appropriate wavelength.

15: Jablonski diagram showing photo-excitation and possible transitions in a molecule.[1]

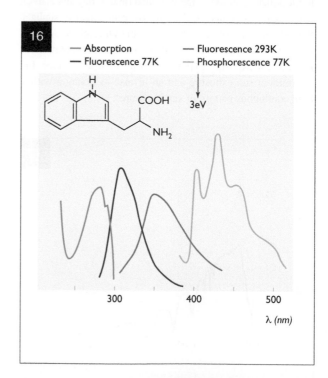

16: Absorption, fluorescence and phosphorescence spectra of a molecule (tryptophan). The fluorescence and phosphorescence spectra appear at longer wavelengths (lower photon energy) than absorption.[1]

If the molecule is in an excited singlet state, the outer electron may be more easily removed, leading to photo-ionization. This is more likely at shorter wavelengths (<300 nm) because of the higher photon energy. Although ionization may not occur, it is nonetheless true that the excited molecule has a different electronic configuration compared with the ground state, and is often able to form a complex with another species. Any photochemical process in which there is a transfer of reactivity to a species other than that absorbing the radiation initially is called a photosensitization reaction. Excited triplet states are most likely to be involved, partly as a result of the long lifetime. Oxygen, which has a ground triplet state, is spin-matched with a molecule in an excited triplet state. It is also a good scavenger of free radicals. There are two mechanisms of photo-oxidation (17). In the Type I reaction, the excited sensitizer (singlet or triplet) undergoes a reaction with the substrate or solvent to produce radicals (neutral or ions), which react with oxygen to produce oxygenated products. In the Type II process, the excited sensitizer reacts with oxygen to form singlet molecular oxygen which then reacts with the substrate to form the oxygenated products. The Type II reaction involves electronic energy transfer from the excited triplet photosensitizer to spin-matched ground state molecular oxygen, returning the sensitizer to the ground state (that is, photosensitizer regeneration).

Action spectrum

The action spectrum is a measure of the importance of each wavelength in producing a particular photobiologic response. It is obtained by measuring the radiation dose required to evoke a particular response at different wavelengths. To plot the action spectrum, make a graph of the reciprocal of the required dose against wavelength. Constructing an action spectrum is an important tool in the investigation of normal and abnormal responses of the skin to UV radiation. Ideally, an action spectrum should resemble the absorption spectrum of the chromophore responsible for the process. This holds for simple systems such as bacteria where DNA was identified as the main chromophore for inactivation. In more complex systems like skin, interference from other molecules and the optical properties of the tissue make interpretation of action spectra more complicated. The so-called SCUP-m action spectrum for UV-carcinogenesis in hairless mice shows a maximum at 293 nm. Applying a correction factor to allow for the difference in optical transmission between mouse and human skin permits extrapolation to humans, the SCUP-h action spectrum. This is shown along with a standard erythemal action spectrum in 18.

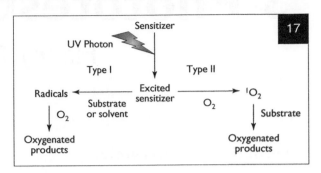

17: Type I and Type II reactions.[2]
18: Action spectra, SCUP-m, SCUP-h, and the CIE erythema action spectrum.[3]

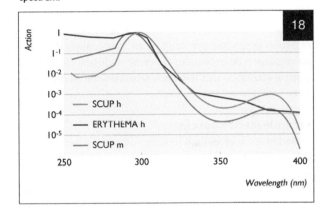

References

1. Kohen E, Santus R, Hirschberg JG. *Photobiology*. San Diego: Academic Press, 1995.

2. Karlsen J. Light-activated drugs and drug formulations in drug targeting. In: *Photostability of Drugs and Drug Formulations:* Tonnesen HH, ed. London: Taylor and Francis, 1996.

3. De Gruil FR, van der Leun JC. Estimate of the wavelength dependency of ultraviolet carcinogenesis in humans and its relevance to the risk assessment of a stratospheric ozone depletion. *Health Physics* 1994;**67**:319–25.

4. Gandini S, Sera F, Cattaruzza MS, Pasquini P, Picconi O, Boyle P, Melchi CF 2005. Meta-analysis of risk factors for cutaneous melanoma: II. Sun exposure. *European Journal of Cancer* **41**: 45-60.

Further reading

Moore DE. Photophysical and photochemical aspects of drug stability. In *Photostability of Drugs and Drug Formulations:* Tonnesen HH, ed. London: Taylor and Francis, 1996.

Young AR. Chromophores in human skin. In : Moseley H, ed. *Optical Radiation Techniques in Medicine and Biology, Phys Med Biol* 1997;**42**: (special issue) 789–802.

3 Phototest Equipment
Harry Moseley

Production of ultraviolet (UV) emission

There are two basic mechanisms of UV emission. One is the process of incandescence whereby a substance emits radiation depending primarily on its temperature; the other accompanies de-excitation, whereby radiation is emitted when a substance that has been raised into an excited state drops into a lower energy level.

Incandescent sources

Incandescent sources emit light by virtue of the fact that they are hot. The best known example of this is the sun. Radiation from an incandescent source appears as a continuous spectrum. The total amount of radiated power increases with temperature; also, the proportion of short-wavelength emission increases as temperature rises. UV radiation is emitted in significant quantity when temperature exceeds 2500 K (19).

Gas discharge lamps

Basic physical laws describe radiation from a perfect radiator (called a *black body*). Incandescent sources are usually ascribed a certain color temperature, defined as the temperature of a black body that emits the same relative visible spectral distribution as the source. The color temperatures of several common sources are given in *Table 3.1*.

Quartz halogen lamps

Quartz halogen lamps incorporate a tungsten filament and a halogen gas inside a quartz envelope. As they operate at a higher temperature than ordinary tungsten filament lamps, there is a shift in spectral emission towards shorter wavelengths. Output is critically dependent on operating voltage. A quartz halogen lamp may be usefully employed as a standard light source with calibration performed at a national standards laboratory.

Excitation Sources

Another method of producing UV or visible radiation is to pass an electric current through a gas raising the constituent electrons to an excited state. When they return to a lower level, or ground state, radiation at one or more characteristic wavelengths is emitted.

The wavelengths are dependent on the type of gas present in the lamp and appear as spectral lines. The width of the lines and the amount of radiation in the continuum between them depend on the pressure in the lamp. At low pressures, fine lines with little or no continuum are produced. As pressure is increased, the lines broaden and their relative amounts alter. The magnitude of the continuum also increases. In mercury vapor sources (20), almost all of the radiation at low pressure appears at 254 nm; as pressure is increased other wavelengths become evident, in particular at 313, 365, 405, 435 and 545 nm.

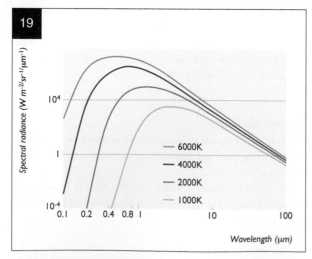

19: Black body spectral radiance.

Table 3.1: Color temperature of various sources

Source	Color temperature (K)
Silicon carbide infrared source	1200
Ordinary tungsten light bulb	2600
Quartz halogen tungsten bulb	3000
Xenon arc lamp	6000
Sun	6000

Arc lamps

These lamps operate at high pressures and are very intense sources of UV radiation. High temperatures are created and broadened spectral lines are superimposed on a continuum arising from the glowing plasma. Commonly available lamps contain xenon, mercury or a mixture of the two elements, and these are all good sources of UV radiation. The *xenon* arc lamp operates at a color temperature of 6000 K and is often used as the light source in a solar simulator or combined with a monochromator in a spectral irradiation system. A delay of approximately 10 minutes is required before the output from a mercury arc lamp is stabilized. Xenon arc lamps do not require a long warm-up period because the xenon is in a gaseous state when the lamp is cold.

In the *carbon* arc lamp (which was widely employed in early phototherapy), an electric discharge is established between two carbon electrodes in air.

The *deuterium* arc lamp provides a useful source of short-wavelength UV radiation. "Point" deuterium arc lamps are available with source diameter of only 1 mm. These may be calibrated at a national standards laboratory and used as a standard reference source. The output of a 50 W deuterium lamp with a fused silica window is similar to that of a 150 W xenon lamp at a wavelength of 200 nm, but the visible radiation content is much less, being only about 0.3% of that of the xenon lamp.

Metal halide lamps

The addition of other metallic elements to a mercury discharge lamp allows for the addition of extra lines to the mercury spectrum. Unfortunately other metals are not sufficiently volatile and also attack the silica envelope. The solution is to introduce the extra metal in halide form (**21**). Most such sources are basically medium pressure mercury discharge lamps with one or more metal halide additives. Advantage has been taken of the strong lead emission lines at 364, 368 and 406 nm in the lead halide lamp where there is a 50% increase in output in the region between 355 and 380 nm compared with a conventional mercury lamp. Antimony and magnesium halide lamps provide spectral lines in the UVB and UVC regions.

Fluorescent lamps

The primary source of radiation in a fluorescent lamp arises from a low-pressure mercury discharge. This produces a strong emission at 254 nm. Clear-walled tubes emit radiation at this wavelength and are used for germicidal purposes, but, strictly speaking, these are not fluorescent lamps. In fluorescent lamps a phosphor coating is applied to the inner wall. The 254 nm radiation produced by the mercury discharge is absorbed in the phosphor coating, where it excites the molecules, causing a fluorescent emission to take place. The output is thus chiefly the fluorescent emission spectrum from the coating with a certain amount of breakthrough of the mercury lines.

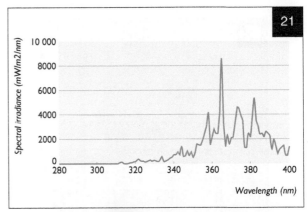

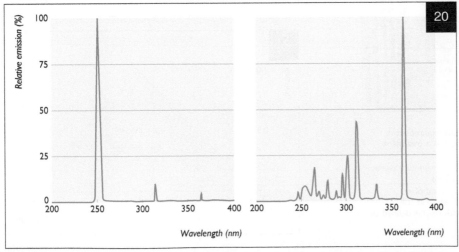

20: Spectral emission from (left) low-pressure and (right) medium-pressure mercury lamp.

21: Output from metal halide lamp.

Phototherapy units

Phototherapy or photochemotherapy is conveniently given in a treatment unit in which the patient is surrounded by UV-emitting lamps. Usually these are fluorescent lamps, but some treatment cabins use metal halide lamps. These units may contain over 50 lamps and so they require high current single-phase or three-phase electrical supply and efficient air-conditioning. Typical units are shown in **22** and the output of commonly used lamps in **23**. Some cabins have built-in sensors but these are not readily adjustable and cannot be assumed to perform accurately or consistently over time. They should not be relied on and should be checked regularly using a hand-held meter.

It is useful to have a small unit available for determining the minimal erythema dose (MED). If this is performed prior to photo (chemo) therapy, it is essential to use the same type of lamps as in the whole-body treatment cabin. The same small unit may be used for hand and foot phototherapy.

Monochromator

A monochromator is a device that disperses light into its constituent wavelengths. The light that emerges from a monochromator has a narrow bandwidth centered at a particular wavelength, which is continuously variable and selectable by the user. The key component in the monochromator is the diffraction grating, which functions like a prism. The grating has very fine etched lines and the light that is reflected off the grating is separated into different wavelengths at different emergent angles. The user selects the desired wavelength by adjusting the angle of the grating. Light enters and exits the device through narrow slits, and the bandwidth is varied by adjusting the slit widths. The radiation throughput depends on the square of the bandwidth. Provided entrance and exit slits are of equal width, a triangular band-pass function is produced (**24**). There is often confusion regarding the definition of bandwidth. It is not appropriate to specify the base of the triangle shown in **24** because monochromators in practice produce a band-pass function with wings that extend out to wavelengths far removed from the center. Because of this,

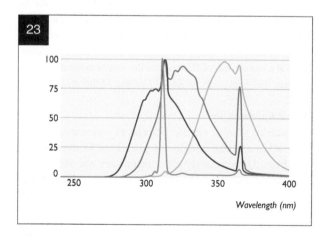

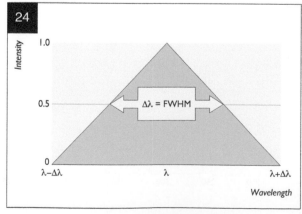

22: A wide range of phototherapy equipment is commercially available. Shown here is a treatment cabin manufactured by Waldmann.

23: Spectral output from commonly-used fluorescent therapy lamps (from Taylor et al 2002).

24: Triangular band-pass function typical of a monochromator, showing the full width at half maximum (FWHM). The bandwidth ($\Delta\lambda$) is defined to be equal to FWHM.

bandwidth is best defined as the full width at half maximum (FWHM), i.e. between the 50% peak intensity points. To avoid confusion, this should be stated explicitly.

In some monochromators, spectral purity is improved by the use of two gratings, so that light emerging from the first grating is incident on a second grating before leaving the monochromator. A monochromator may be used as part of an irradiation system or as part of the measurement system.

Irradiation monochromator

In an irradiation monochromator, light from a xenon arc lamp is coupled to the monochromator and the patient's skin is exposed to "monochromatic" radiation at the selected wavelength and for the desired dose (**25**). It is possible with this device to determine the dose required to produce an outcome, such as an erythema, at a variety of wavelengths. This is particularly useful when testing patients with suspected photodermatosis.

Spectroradiometer

The monochromator is the central unit in a spectroradiometer (see **28**). This is a device for measuring the spectrum, wavelength by wavelength, from a UV source. Light is incident on input optics, which contain a light-scattering element, either a diffuser or an integrating sphere, and enters a monochromator. The light emerging from the exit slit of the monochromator is measured by a detector, usually a photomultiplier tube. Most modern spectroradiometers are computer controlled with wavelength change carried out using a stepping motor.

UV detectors

The conventional UV detector contains the following components: diffuser, filter, sensor, display and associated electronics (**26**). The diffuser is required, otherwise light measurement will be strongly dependent on the angle between the source and the face of the detector. This can be a significant source of error, particularly when the detector is used to measure UV radiation from large sources, such as a 1.8 m UV fluorescent lamp. Next, the filter transmits the wavelengths that are to be measured by the sensor. The response of the detector at different wavelengths depends on both the filter and the sensor. Most detectors use a photodiode as the sensor. Essentially, a photodiode produces an electrical current on exposure to UV or visible radiation. The signal is then amplified and displayed on a digital scale.

Since the UV detector is the device that measures the dose to the patient, there should be careful consideration given to its selection. For a PUVA meter, wavelength response should be predominantly UVA (315–400 nm); for a UVB meter it should be predominantly UVB (280–315 nm). Angular response should ideally be cosine (f2 error as defined in CIE69 should not exceed 10%). Dynamic range should be 0.1 mW/cm² to 50 mW/cm². It should be calibrated, traceable to a national standard, easy to use, low temperature coefficient, robust, lightweight and portable. Cost is the final consideration.

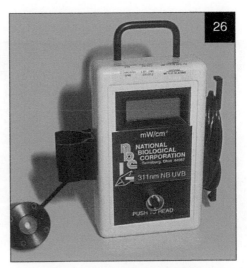

25: Irradiation monochromator (left) used to test patient sensitivity at discrete wavelengths; erythemal response (right) is observed 24 hours later.

26: UV detector based on a filtered photodiode.

Thermopiles

The thermopile operates on a different principle from the photodiode. Light is absorbed on a blackened surface and the associated temperature rise is measured by a series of thermocouples (**27**). It has a flat spectral response over a broad range of wavelengths, which makes it ideal for use with an irradiation monochromator. However, thermopiles are not as sensitive as photodiodes. Also, they must be used with care, since it is the difference between the temperature of the blackened target and a reference point on the device that is measured. So they are susceptible to variations in environmental temperature and drafts. They are generally more fragile than photodiodes.

Calibration

Every UV detector used in a phototherapy unit should be regularly calibrated (**28**). The calibration method should be appropriate to the detector. A frequency of once per year is usually acceptable. Calibration helps to ensure that patients receive the required dose that is important for optimal outcome. Moreover, if a patient is burnt during a course of treatment, then in the event of litigation, the responsible clinician will be expected to know the dose that the patient received.

If the unit has a spectroradiometer for measurement of spectra, this may be calibrated using lamps that have been calibrated at a primary standards calibration laboratory (for example, the National Physical Laboratory). This is costly but necessary.

All units will have access to PUVA or UVB meters. These can only be calibrated properly using a spectroradiometer. The technique is as follows:

1 Measure the spectral irradiance from the appropriate light source using a calibrated spectroradiometer.
2 Sum the spectral irradiances across the waveband of interest.
3 Place the entrance aperture of the sensor at the same point as the input optics of the spectroradiometer and note the reading.
4 Adjust the meter display so that it reads the irradiance determined spectroradiometrically.

If the unit possesses a thermopile this should be calibrated by a primary standards laboratory.

Comparison checks should be carried out regularly (for example, monthly) in between the annual absolute calibrations. All results should be documented so that if one meter or one lamp begins to drift in its performance, this will be easily identified.

Comparison of UV lamps for phototesting

Considering the variety of lamps available, the pros and cons of different lamps used for phototesting are summarized in *Table 3.2*.

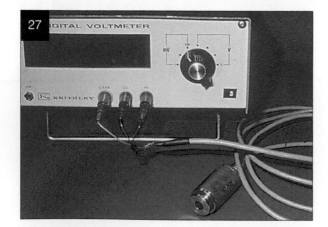

27: Thermopile detects the temperature rise when light is incident on a blackened surface.

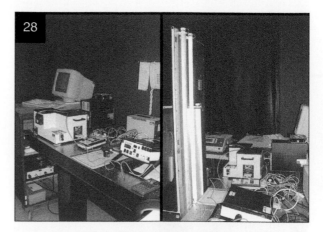

28: Spectroradiometer used to measure the spectral irradiance from a UV source during a routine detector calibration.

Scottish UltraViolet Dosimetry Guidelines: "ScUViDo"

Dosimetry guidelines, known as "ScUViDo", were drawn up by a group of dermatologists and physicists working in Scotland. The aim was to ensure consistency in dose measurements for patients undergoing PUVA or narrowband (TL-01) UVB therapy in centers throughout Scotland. Dosimetry in many centers outside Scotland is based on these or an earlier version of the Scottish Guidelines. They are deliberately descriptive rather than prescriptive,

Table 3.2: **Comparison of UV lamps for phototesting**

Fluorescent lamps
   Advantages
   • Same spectrum as the treatment
   • Large area for provocation
   Disadvantages
   • Lamp size may be inconvenient
   • Fixed spectrum

Metal halide lamps
   Advantages
   • High UVA content
   • Useful for provocation
   Disadvantages
   • Broad range of lamp types with different spectra
   • Non-uniform distribution over area

Solar simulator
   Advantages
   • Rapid screening for photosensitivity
   • Beam area suitable for provocation
   Disadvantages
   • Spectrum varies with each instrument
   • MED dependent on choice of cut-off filters
   • Moderately expensive

Irradiation monochromator
   Advantages
   • Well-defined selectable spectrum
   • Essential for diagnosis of type of photodermatosis
   Disadvantages
   • Small irradiation area
   • Time-consuming
   • Requires skilled staff
   • Expensive

emphasizing the importance of understanding the principles rather than blindly applying a methodology.

Meter calibration

The meter should be calibrated against a bank of fluorescent lamps similar in spectral emission to those used in the treatment unit. A PUVA meter should be calibrated using appropriate UVA lamps, and similarly for narrowband (TL01) or broadband UVB meter. The spectral irradiance from the fluorescent lamps should be measured using a calibrated spectroradiometer. For PUVA lamps the UVA component (315–400 nm) should be determined. For UVB lamps, the UVB dose should be quoted or the total UV (UVA + UVB) if the user prefers to use this. Although the action spectrum for clearance of psoriasis has not been fully defined, published data are strongly suggestive that wavelengths around 311 nm are optimal, and so quoting UVB would seem to be appropriate. It should be clearly stated whether calibration is given for UVB or total UV.

Designated patient irradiance

An important principle is that dosimetry should be patient based (**29**). To this end, designated patient irradiance (DPI) is defined as the mean irradiance incident on a subject of average height and build in a treatment unit at chest, waist and knee level. At each level, irradiance should be measured on the anterior, posterior, right and left surfaces. The DPI may be measured by the direct or indirect method.

Direct method

For this method, the investigator measures the irradiance at the specified body sites, while standing in the treatment unit. The mean irradiance of the body sites gives the DPI directly. This measures the dose received by the patient directly.

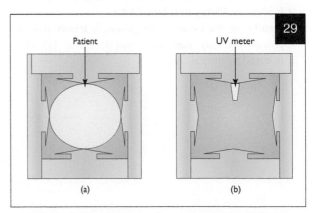

29: Diagram showing (a) patient in UV cabin compared with (b) UV meter in an empty cabin. The meter receives reflected radiation from lamps on opposite side. This is a potential source of error.

Indirect method

An alternative method is to measure the irradiance from each bank of lamps in a standard manner, clamping the detector in a support. This is, arguably, more reproducible than the direct method and allows measurements to be made without the danger of exposure of the investigator. However, it is necessary to apply a correction factor because the mean irradiance with the unit unoccupied is not equal to the DPI. So, it would be appropriate to measure the DPI initially using the direct method. At the same time, measurements may be taken using the indirect method so that a correction factor may be calculated. Reproducibility should be within ±10%.

In-built dosimetry

Some treatment cabins have in-built sensors designed to monitor the UV dose to the patient. Unfortunately, these have been found to be very unreliable. Patient times should be calculated from the measurements made according to the dosimetry guidelines.

Safety

Ultraviolet radiation is potentially harmful. Staff should exercise prudent avoidance to ensure that eyes and skin are not exposed unnecessarily to UV radiation from treatment sources. Face masks, goggles, sunscreen and protective suits should be provided and used as appropriate (**30**).

The importance of dosimetry

Accurate and reproducible dosimetry underpins a scientific approach to photodermatology. It is important for the following reasons.

- It facilitates safe and effective patient care.
- It permits safe transfer of patient from one center to another.
- It allows for staff movement to new centers.
- It gives credibility to published data.
- Finally, in the event of litigation, it means that the practitioner may state with confidence the UV dose received by the patient.

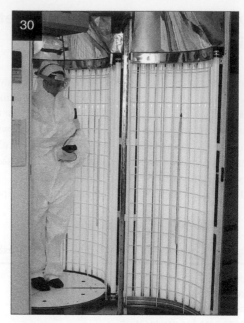

30: UV protective clothing and eyewear being used during direct measurements of UV incident on a subject in the treatment unit.

References

1. Taylor DK, Austey AV, Coleman AJ, et al. Guidelines for dosimetry and calibration in ultraviolet radiation therapy: a report of a British Photodermatology Group workshop. Br J Dermatol 2002;**146**:755–63.

Further reading

Boyd RW. *Radiometry and the Detection of Optical Radiation.* New York: John Wiley & Sons, 1983.

Diffey BL, Hart G. *Ultraviolet and Blue-Light Phototherapy – Principals, Source, Dosimetry and Safety.* York: The Institute of Physics and Engineering in Medicine, 1997.

Moseley H. *Non-Ionising Radiation.* Bristol: Adam Hilger Publications, 1988.

Moseley H. Scottish UV Dosimetry Guidelines, "ScUViDo". *Photodermatol Photoimmunol Photomed* 2001;**17**: 30–33.

4 Photoprotection
Harry Moseley

There are essentially three components to a photoprotection strategy; these are, in order of priority: behavior, clothing, and sunscreens. Appropriate behavior avoids the problem; wearing suitable clothing provides a continuous barrier to covered areas; use of sunscreens is designed to protect the skin by application of a surface chemical optical filter. Unfortunately, the general public tend to rank these three components in reverse order with sunscreens being the primary source of photoprotection. There are many reasons for this – advertising, the pleasant feeling (for some) of sun on skin, the desire for personal freedom of action. The patient with a photo-induced skin disorder has generally learned from bitter experience to adopt the recommended ranking order of behavior, clothing, and sunscreens.

UV index

It is useful to know how much UV radiation there is from sunlight at any particular location and this is often reported in the media or on various websites as a UV Index (UVI). This is a measure of the intensity of UV radiation on the earth's surface. Its use is endorsed by the World Health Organization to raise public awareness and alert people to the need for adopting protective measures. The higher the index value, the greater the potential for damage to skin and eye. UVI is defined by the equation:

$$UVI = k \bullet IE_\lambda \, S_{er} = (\lambda) \, d\lambda$$

where E_λ is the solar spectral irradiance (W/m²/nm) and S_{er} (λ) is the standard CIE erythema action spectrum;[1] k is simply a constant (set at 40 m²/W) that scales the erythema-weighted solar spectral irradiance to a simple whole number, usually between 1 and 10.

Behavioral changes for sun avoidance

In countries where there are high levels of sunlight, behavioral changes can make a major contribution to UV reduction in personal exposure. For example, in Australia taking advantage of times when solar UV is low (avoid 4 hours around solar noon) and using shade (providing additional 50% protection) can reduce personal exposure by a factor of 10.

Sun characteristics
UV radiation levels are influenced by a number of factors and it is useful to summarize these to inform a sun avoidance strategy.

Sun elevation
UV radiation is attenuated as the sun's rays pass through the earth's atmosphere. The path length through the atmosphere is determined by the elevation of the sun. Hence UV radiation varies with the time of day. Approximately 60% of the total UV during a summer's day is incident in the 4-hour period around solar noon (which may be 13.00 local time). Also, for the same reason, it varies with the time of year.

Latitude
UV radiation increases with proximity to the equator.

Cloud cover
Clouds attenuate UV radiation to a highly variable degree. Over 90% of UV can penetrate light cloud but dense cloud can reduce UV levels by a factor of 6.

Altitude
Although the main attenuation of UVB occurs in the stratosphere about 19–23 km above the surface of the earth, attenuation also occurs nearer the ground. This means that UV radiation levels increase with altitude. With every 1000 meters, UV rises by 10–12%.

On reflection
In addition to UV radiation incident direct, it is also important to consider reflection from various surfaces. This can be as much as 80% from fresh snow, 25% from sand and 15% from smooth sea. Water, however, transmits UV radiation to the extent that at half a meter depth, UV is still 40% as intense as at the surface.

Shade

Shade removes UV radiation directly from the sun but UV radiation scattered from the sky is not excluded. The degree of protection depends on the amount of sky that can be seen within the shaded area. As a rule of thumb, shade can reduce UV radiation by approximately 50%. However, in these circumstances it is important to recognize that 2 hours in shade is equivalent to 1 hour in sunlight. It is misleading to assume that the attenuation of the material corresponds to the protection afforded by the structure. Trees can provide natural shade but the extent of cover depends on the canopy provided by the leaves and the branches.

Windows

Window glass effectively absorbs the UVB component from sunlight. Transmission is approximately 0.2% for 4 mm thickness and 0.004% for double glazing. However, UVA is transmitted quite effectively (31). Response of a patient to sunlight through window glass may therefore indicate whether there is an abnormal sensitivity to UVA, which might be masked by the normal UVB erythemal response.

Blinds

The use of plastic blinds to provide protection from UV and visible light below 470 nm has been found helpful in the management of patients with severe photodermatoses. Blinds constructed from a UV-attenuating material, such as the yellow material Uvethon Y, fixed to the ward roof may be raised or lowered as required.

Self-adhesive window film can be applied to the windows in the people's homes. There are several suppliers of suitable materials, which give good UV protection, and some of these are listed in *Table 4.1*.

Clothing

The use of clothing and hats is the next step after sun avoidance in a practical photoprotection strategy. Clothing does not suffer from the uncertainties that apply to sunscreen use. It is fairly obvious which parts of the body are covered and the level of protection does not change during the course of the day, provided the material is kept dry.

Ultraviolet protection factor (UPF)

Australia and New Zealand were the first countries to introduce a product standard for garments claiming to provide UV protection. The degree of protection is determined by the UPF, which is analogous to the sun protection factor used for sunscreens. UPF is generally measured *in vitro* by recording the UV transmittance, which is then applied to the sunlight spectrum and erythema action spectrum to compute the level of protection afforded by the fabric.

The Australian Radiation Laboratory pioneered the swing tag UPF rating with the protection message on the reverse side (32). Clothing has been specially developed particularly designed for children (33). The level of protection afforded by clothing depends on several factors.[2]

Weave

The weave is the most important factor affecting the transmission of UV radiation. The more closely woven a fabric is, the less UV radiation is transmitted. Most of the UV penetration through fabrics takes place through the spaces between the yarns. Spaces between the yarns are generally larger in a knit fabric than in a woven textile.

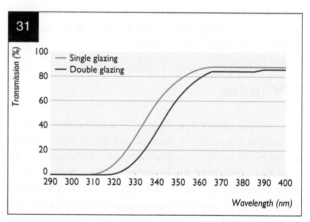

31: Transmission through samples of window glass.

Table 4.1: Window films that absorb UV radiation

Product	Manufacturer/Supplier
DermaGard	Sun-Gard, Florida, USA Bonwyke Window Films, Fareham, Hampshire, UK
Llumar Window Films CourtGard	CPFilms Inc, Martinsville, Virginia, USA
GlassGard	Film Technologies International Inc, St Petersburg, Florida, USA
ScotchTint	3M Energy Products Distribution, Baltimore, MD, USA

Colour

The absorption band of dyes often extends into the UV region so that fabrics that are dark in colour also exhibit higher UV absorption, thus increasing the UPF.

Weight

The weight of a material is also a factor. Provided weave and color are identical, a weightier fabric implies more material and so higher UV absorption.

Stretch

Fabrics such as elastane and Lycra can be stretched and the amount of UV transmission is highly dependent on the degree of stretch. The UPF of elastane is reduced by approximately 50% when stretched by 10%. The most popular type of stockings (15 denier) provides a UPF of <2, which is further reduced on stretching.

Surgical gloves are often used to provide occupational UV protection and these are generally suitable for this purpose. Although transmission doubled when stretched, all types tested were acceptable apart from one type, called Tru-Touch, which gave 7.32 ± 1.49% UVA transmission when tested under stretch conditions.

Water

The effect of water on UV transmission depends on the fabric. The presence of water in the spaces of a fabric reduces optical scattering. In the case of cotton T-shirts when wet, the UPF drops to about half the dry value. This is important when these items of clothing are being worn on the beach, as children are often in and out of the water during play.

Washing

The UPF of cotton or polyester/cotton garments increases significantly after the first wash. One study reported a mean UPF of 20.2 ± 2.5 when new, which increased to 38.3 ± 4.2 after one wash, and was 39.9 ± 3.1 after 36 washes. Most fabrics undergo a combination of relaxation and shrinkage that reduces the spaces between the yarns.

UV absorbers

UV absorbers for laundry detergents and rinse cycle have been developed. Application of UV absorbers significantly enhances the UV protection of a garment, especially that of non-dyed lightweight summer fabrics, which are intrinsically low.

Conclusion

Clothing can provide significant protection against solar UV radiation. UPF values for cotton or polyester/cotton range between 7 and >100. Light-sensitive individuals should be careful regarding the amount of protection afforded by light

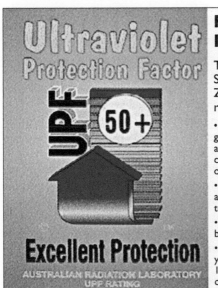

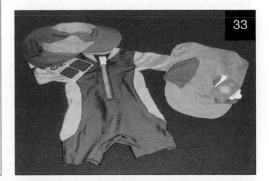

32: A swing tag used to designate UPF rating on clothing. It refers to the AS/NZS 4399 (1996) Sun Protective Clothing Standard and has a message on the back from the Australian and New Zealand Cancer Societies. (courtesy of Peter Gies).

33: Examples of high UPF children's clothing manufactured from Lycra.

clothing. Lycra is lightweight with good protection. General recommendations are listed in *Table 4.2*. It is important to emphasize that UPF is based on the normal erythemal action spectrum and is therefore dominated by UVB radiation absorption. Many fabrics transmit significant amounts of UVA, which may provoke a reaction in photosensitive patients.

Sunscreens

The last line in a photoprotection strategy is the use of topical sunscreens. In the eyes of the general public, however, sunscreens tend to top the list of sun protection measures. This is due in part to the way in which sunscreens are marketed. Cosmetic sun products were initially designed to be tanning aids promoted by Coco Chanel in the 1930s. The transformation from tan enhancing to sun protection products took place some 40 years later, and the concept of the sun protective factor emerged. This was developed to indicate the level of protection from burning afforded by the product. Eventually the short-comings of this index were realized and the industry responded with other indicators of performance, particularly with regard to protection against the effects of skin aging caused by UVA irradiation.

Active ingredients

The active ingredients in topical sunscreens are usually divided into chemical and physical compounds. Chemical, organic sunscreens absorb over relatively narrow wavebands, mainly in the UVB but nowadays also extending into the UVA *(Table 4.3)*. Physical sunscreens are inorganic substances that reflect and scatter both UV and visible radiation.

In chemical sunscreens, UV radiation is traditionally absorbed by the alternating single and double bonds in heterocyclic rings (for example, Eusolex 8020, Parsol 1789). These structures may also undergo photochemical trans-formation and cause phototoxic and photo-allergic reactions. Sixteen UV absorbers were approved in Europe in 1996, the most common being octyl-methoxycinnamate, methyl-benzylidene camphor, phenylbenzimidazole sulfonic acid, isoamyl p-methylcinnamate, octyl-dimethyl PABA, PEG-25 PABA, and octyltriazone. PABA (p-aminobenzoic acid), also known as vitamin H, and its derivatives are rarely used. Sunscreens usually contain lipophilic and hydrophilic absorbers. There are also four UVA absorbers approved in Europe. One of these, Mexoryl SX, was developed by L'Oreal and has been on the market since 1991. Its maximum absorption is at 345 nm.

Table 4.2: **Significance of various factors with respect to UV protective clothing**

Factor	Significance
Fabric material	Polyester – high UPF; nylon, wool and silk – moderate UPF; cotton, viscose, rayon and silk – low UPF
Porosity	Next to fabric material in importance
Color	Darker colors have higher UPF
Transparency	Less transparent higher UPF
UV absorbers	Increase UPF
Stretch	Decreases UPF
Wetness	Decreases UPF (especially cotton)
Washing	Increases UPF (especially cotton)
Cover	The garment should cover the skin as much as possible
Fit	Loose fit is preferable
UVA	UVA transmission may be significant

Physical sunscreens generally provide broad-spectrum protection using substances such as microfine titanium dioxide. They have the advantage that they have no photosensitizing properties, and are often used in conjunction with chemical absorbers. Both titanium dioxide and zinc oxide have been approved as sunscreens. The efficiency is not as high as that of organic filters, and high concentrations are required for high protection. Pigmentary titanium dioxide with a particle size above 200 nm has its greatest efficiency to visible radiation and causes whitening of the skin, which may be cosmetically undesirable. On the other hand if the particle size is micronized to below 100 nm, efficiency shifts to the UV and skin whitening is reduced. Special sunscreens designed for sensitive skin usually contain physical substances and exclude chemical absorbers, preservatives, and fragrance.

Sun protection factor

The sun protection factor (SPF) is the ratio of the dose of UV radiation that causes a minimal erythema in unprotected skin to that which causes a minimal erythema in skin protected by the sunscreen. For example, if the normal MED is 30 mJ/cm^2

Table 4.3: **Properties of organic filters used in sunscreens**[6]

General class	Organic filter	Wavelength of max. absorption	Class of sunscreen	EC approved	US approved
PABA derivative	PABA aminobenzoic acid	283 nm	UVB	Yes	Yes
PABA derivative	Octyl-dimethyl PABA	311, 300 nm	UVB	Yes	Yes
Methoxycinnamate ester	Octyl-methoxycinna-mate	289, 311 nm	UVB	Yes	Yes
Methoxycinnamate ester	Isopentyl-methoxycinnamate	308 nm	UVB	Yes	No
Methoxycinnamate ester	Diethanolamine methoxycinnamate	290 nm	UVB	No	Yes
Salicylate ester	Homomenthyl salicylate	306, 308 nm	UVB	Yes	Yes
Salicylate ester	Octyl-salicylate	307, 310 nm	UVB	Yes	Yes
Salicylate ester	Triethanolamine salicylate	298 nm	UVB	No	Yes
Benzophenone	Benzophenone-3	288, 325, 329 nm	UVA	Yes	Yes
Benzophenone	Benzophenone-4	286, 324 nm	UVA	Yes	Yes
Benzophenone	Benzophenone-8	284, 327, 296, 352 nm	UVA	No	Yes
Dibenzoylmethanes	Butyl-methoxy-dibenzoylmethanes	358 nm	UVA	Yes	No
Dibenzoylmethanes	4-isopropyl-diben-zoylmethanes	345 nm	UVA	Yes	No

and the MED of the protected skin is 450 mJ/cm^2, the SPF is 15. In other words, application of the sunscreen has caused an increase by a factor of 15 in the dose required to induce erythema. It must be emphasized that SPF refers to protection against UV-induced erythema. Extrapolation to other harmful effects is extremely problematic and could be quite misleading. It is principally a measure of the UVB attenuation of the sunscreen. According to the test methods adopted by most manufacturers, the UVB component of the light source used contributes 85% of the total erythema.

Although conceptually very simple, it is often misunderstood by the general public, who imagine that use of a high factor sunscreen will protect them against the harmful effects of UV radiation. Even if the sunscreen provides the protection indicated by the SPF, a day's exposure outdoors wearing a factor 15 sunscreen will still result in more than an MED for many individuals. This misconception often leads individuals to stay in the sun longer than they should. There is also a major difference between the highly controlled conditions in the

Table 4.4: **Factors influencing SPF variability* (Brown M, personal communication)**

Factors	Standard SPF test	In-use situation	Effect on in-use SPF
Thickness of application	2.0 mg/cm^2	0.5–1.5 mg/cm^2	REDUCED SPF
Spreading and rubbing in	Controlled even spreading, by trained technician	Uneven spreading and variable run-in procedure	REDUCED SPF
Substantivity	No possibility of product removal	Loss of product due to wash-off, rub-off, and so on, highly likely	REDUCED SPF
Angle of incidence of UV exposure	90° incident	Variable incidence. Effectively increasing path length through sunscreen	INCREASED SPF

sunscreen laboratory and outdoor real-life product use. Some of these are listed in *Table 4.4* and the overall effect is to significantly reduce the actual SPF experienced in practice.

Several standard methodologies have been developed, notably in Germany, Japan, South Africa, USA, and Australia. A European standard (COLIPA) is now in widespread use in several countries and some of the previous anomalies are disappearing as harmonization gains pace.

Thickness of application

The SPF is determined based on a uniform application thickness of 2 mg/cm^2. In practice, however, only between 0.5 and 1.5 mg/cm^2 is used,[3] principally because of the high cost of sunscreen. The effect of application thickness is shown diagrammatically in **34** for the ideal scenario of uniform application. This demonstrates how light absorption depends strongly on thickness. For example, a sunscreen labeled SPF 16 is reduced to an SPF of 2 if the consumer applies 0.5 mg/cm^2.

Another related factor is that of uniformity of application. The manufacturers take considerable care when applying the sunscreen, using trained staff spreading with a gloved finger. This is not the way that sunscreen is used in practice, and areas such as tops of ears may be skipped. The same amount of sunscreen non-uniformly applied implies that some areas receive little or no sunscreen. This means that large areas of skin have little or no protection and so the effective SPF is reduced even further. Where the sunscreen has been applied, there may well be virtually total protection but there will still be areas of skin more or less exposed to the direct sunlight.

Substantivity

During the course of the day, sunscreen is removed from the skin by water, sweat, toweling, clothing, and sand. Most commercially available sunscreens now claim to be water resistant with some also claiming to be rub resistant and sand resistant. Consumers are often encouraged to re-apply sunscreen regularly. This not only replaces the sunscreen that has been removed by water or rubbing but also helps to ensure sufficient application, given that most people significantly under-apply in the first place.

Water-resistance testing is only standardized in the USA and Australia, where SPF is assessed after a bathing period of 40 minutes. Other test procedures include forming a stream of water that flows evenly over the test area at a standardized water temperature, flow rate, and watering time.

Beyond the SPF

As sunscreens evolved to provide protection from UVA as well as UVB radiation, it soon became clear that a parameter had to be developed to label UVA protection. Boots Group PLC led the way with their "UVA star rating system" *(Table 4.5)*. Four stars indicate that the product offers a balanced amount of UVA and UVB protection; a three, two or one star rating indicates decreasing UVA protection. In the absence of an agreed industry standard, other manufacturers developed their own labeling system. Another technique involves the critical wavelength determination. In this method, the critical wavelength occurs where 90% of the area under the absorbance versus wavelength curve occurs. A product with high critical wavelength extends the protection out to longer wavelengths and therefore provides more UVA protection. The term "sunblock" has recently appeared and generally refers to a product that provides high SPF (at least 25) and good UVA protection. The phrase "total sunblock" should be avoided as this implies a complete absence of UV penetration to the skin.

There is no general acceptance on how to evaluate UVA protection. Many investigators have used immediate pigment darkening (IPD) or permanent pigment darkening (PPD) as the endpoint, while others have relied on *in vitro* methods. Needless to say, the results are not comparable.

Antioxidants may also have a role in skin care, particularly in reduction of epidermal lipid peroxidation and prevention of DNA damage. They may also provide protection from sunburn. Some manufacturers are including antioxidants or free radical scavengers in their sunscreens and labeling them as such.

In recent years the number of variants on the market has increased dramatically with specialist products for children, teenagers, sensitive skin, sports use, and products where protection is incorporated in insect protection, moisturizers, make-up foundations and lipsticks.[5]

Sunscreens for photosensitive patients

Many patients suffering from a photodermatosis use sunscreens to provide photoprotection. Some are sensitive to visible as well as UV radiation. Unfortunately, commercial sunscreens are formulated to confer protection against UV radiation with little or no protection in the visible region,

particularly as this would impact on the color of the product. In order to extend protection into the UVA region, products have been developed with microfine titanium dioxide and zinc oxide particles. The small particle size enhances cosmetic acceptability but reduces reflection (and hence protection) of visible radiation.

Commercial sunscreens were tested on patients with chronic actinic dermatitis using UV radiation at 300, 350, and 400 nm. They gave high protection at 300 nm (up to 55 protection factor), less at 350 nm, and very little at 400 nm (protection factor 2).

A small range of reflectant sunscreens using larger particle size (pigment grade) titanium dioxide and zinc oxide was developed to provide extra protection for patients with photosensitivity extending into the visible region of the spectrum.[4] Transmission of several sunscreens in the UV and visible region is shown in **35**. Since the normal SPF is of little

Table 4.5: **UVA star rating system indicates the relative UVA protection compared to UVB. Four stars indicates equivalent protection from UVA and UVB. For proper interpretation, it must be used in conjunction with the SPF**

UVA/UVB absorption ratio	Star rating
0.00–0.19	No rating
0.20–0.39	*
0.40–0.59	**
0.60–0.79	***
0.80–1.00	****

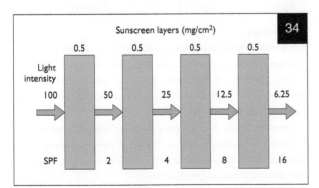

34: Diagram to illustrate the effect of applying a reduced amount of sunscreen. In the example, each layer has a thickness equivalent to 0.5 mg/cm², which reduces the relevant light intensity by a factor of 2. Four layers, equivalent to 2.0 mg/cm², reduces the relative light intensity from 100 to 6.25, which corresponds to an SPF of 16. However, if only 0.5 mg/cm² is applied, relative light intensity is reduced from 100 to 50, an SPF of only 2!

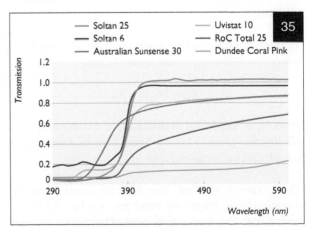

35: Transmission of commercially available sunscreens showing the low level of attenuation in the visible part of the spectrum (above 390 nm) compared to the sunscreen Dundee Coral Pink, developed to provide protection to patients with photosensitivity in the blue light region.[4]

relevance to patients with one of the photodermatoses, a new index, called the photosensitivity protection factor (PPF), was introduced. The PPF is analogous to the SPF with the normal erythemal action spectrum replaced by the patient's photosensitivity action spectrum, and the sunlight spectrum extended to 600 nm. SPF was not a good indicator of PPF, according to the *in vitro* tests. For example, SPF and PPF values were, respectively, 26 and 2.3 for Soltan 25, and 24 and 2.7 for Australian Sunsense 30. Although the commercial sunscreens had low PPFs, the new products gave much higher PPF levels. For example, Dundee Coral Pink had an SPF of 14 and PPF of 9.6. For the photosensitive patient, it is the PPF that matters. These results were confirmed *in vivo* at 430 nm, where the median protective factor for a group of photosensitive patients using SunE45 (SPF 25) was 2, compared to 8 for one of the new sunscreens (Dundee Beige).

Exposure standards

Occupational exposure standards have been developed to provide guidelines on limits of exposure to ultraviolet radiation and these are widely adopted in many countries.[6]

As regards the unprotected eye, for UVA (315–400 nm), the total radiant exposure should not exceed 10 kJ/cm^2 (1.0 J/cm^2) within an 8-hour period; for UVB and UVC (180–315 nm), the total radiant exposure should not exceed 30 J/m^2 weighted by the factor S_λ given in *Table 4.6*.

For unprotected skin, the total radiant exposure in the spectral region 180–400 nm should not exceed 30 J/m^2 weighted by the factor S_λ.

To determine the effective irradiance (E_{eff}) of a broadband source, the following formula should be used:

$$E_{eff} = \Sigma E_\lambda S_\lambda = \Delta\lambda$$

where E_λ is the spectral irradiance, S_λ is the relative spectral effectiveness given in *Table 4.5*, and $\Delta\lambda$ is the bandwidth of the calculated or measured intervals.

These exposure standards have been developed to prevent unwanted acute effects but these may not be adequate to protect from long-term effects induced by chronic, repeated exposure. Also, it should be noted that these limits do not apply to patient exposure for therapeutic purposes.

Table 4.6: **Occupational UV radiation exposure limits and spectral weighting function**[5]

Wavelength (nm)	Exposure limit (mJ/cm^2)	Relative spectral effectiveness (S_λ)
180	250	0.012
190	160	0.019
200	100	0.030
205	59	0.051
210	40	0.075
215	32	0.095
220	25	0.120
225	20	0.150
230	16	0.190
235	13	0.240
240	20	0.300
245	8.3	0.360
250	7.0	0.430
255	5.8	0.520
260	4.6	0.650
265	3.7	0.810
270	3.0	1.000
275	3.1	0.960
280	3.4	0.880
285	3.9	0.770
290	4.7	0.640
295	5.6	0.540
300	10	0.300
305	50	0.060
310	200	0.015
315	1.0×10^3	0.003
320	2.9×10^3	0.0010
325	6.0×10^3	0.00050
330	7.3×10^3	0.00041
335	8.8×10^3	0.00034
340	1.1×10^4	0.00028
350	1.5×10^4	0.00020
360	2.3×10^4	0.00013
370	3.2×10^4	0.000093
380	4.7×10^4	0.000064
390	6.8×10^4	0.000044
400	1.0×10^5	0.000030

References

1. International Organization for Standardization. *Erythema Reference Action Spectrum and Standard Erythema Dose.* ISO 17166: 1999.

2. Gies PH, Roy CR, McLennan A. Textiles and sun protection. *In: Environmental UV-Radiation, Risk of Skin Cancer and Primary Prevention.* Stuttgart: Gustav Fischer, 1996.

3. Diffey BL. Has sun protection factor had its day? *BMJ* 2000;**320**:176–7.

4. Moseley H, Cameron H, MacLeod T, Clark C, Dawe R, Ferguson J. New sunscreens confer improved protection for photosensitive patients in the blue light region. *Br J Dermatol* 2001;**145**:789–94.

5. Busick TL, Uchida T, Wagner RF. 2005 Preventing ultraviolet light lip injury: Beachgoer awareness about lip cancer risk factors and lip protection behaviour. *Dermatologic Surgery* **31**: 173-176.

6. IRPA. *Guidelines on Protection against Non-ionizing Radiation.* New York: Pergamon Press, 1990.

5 Polymorphic Light Eruption

Nicholas J Wainwright

Polymorphic light eruption (PLE), a condition provoked by ultraviolet light, is the commonest of the idiopathic photodermatoses. For the most part, these are separable conditions in clinical practice, although areas of overlap are recognized, notably between PLE and actinic prurigo (AP). In the past, some authors have grouped them together as manifestations of so-called "polymorphous light eruption". The term, introduced by Rasch in 1900, appears in the literature in this broader context but also continues to be used synonymously with polymorphic light eruption such that confusion can arise. Other terms, such as Willan's "eczema solare" and "summer prurigo" refer to some of the earliest recorded descriptions of PLE.

Epidemiology

Prevalence

There have been three simple descriptive surveys but as yet no sound cross-sectional population survey. A prevalence of 10% was recorded from entrants to a Boston medical library while a higher figure of 21% was obtained amongst employees of a Swedish pharmaceutical company. A study conducted in England and Australia produced figures of 14.8% and about 5% which confirmed the observation of PLE being commoner away from the equator.[1]

Age of onset

A series from Tayside, Scotland, shows that 62% (1204/1935) (J Ferguson, personal communication) experienced their first symptoms in the first three decades but onset may occur later even in those previously able to bear strong sunlight.

Sex distribution

The ratio of female to male sufferers ranges from 2:1 in a Swedish series to 6.7:1 in a Scottish series, although this may simply reflect a difference in referral patterns.[2]

Heritability

The evidence for a familial tendency is variable, being more highly reported in Scandinavia than in the United Kingdom or United States[2,3]. A questionnaire of 420 adult female twins showed a higher concordance for polymorphic light eruption for monozygotic (0.72) than dizygotic (0.30) twin pairs. Further, the chance of a positive family history of PLE was significantly higher amongst first-degree relatives of twins where at least one had PLE than for unaffected twins. Such results point to a strong genetic effect in line with the observed familial clustering probably in conjunction with environmental factors. Genetic modeling of photosensitivity in families with PLE and AP has estimated the prevalence of a low penetrance PLE susceptibility allele to be about 72% of the UK population. However, clinical PLE is much less prevalent, suggesting that expression is modified by other genes and environmental factors.[4] A strong HLA association in PLE has not been found as compared with AP where 90% have the DR4 allele and 60% the rare DRB1*0407 allele.

Mechanism

The pathogenesis of PLE is as yet unclear, but the most prominent hypothesis for over half a century has been a delayed-type hypersensitivity response to a cutaneous neo-antigen induced in susceptible individuals by sun exposure.[3] Although this antigen has not been identified, the feasibility of such a mechanism gained credence from the observation of PLE appearing after a photo-allergic contact dermatitis reaction to Fentichlor.[5] Other *in vitro* studies have provided further support for the UV induction of endogenous antigens. The similarity in cellular and adhesion molecule responses in PLE to delayed-type hypersensitivity reactions, such as contact allergic dermatitis or the tuberculin reaction, has been demonstrated by immunohistochemical studies. These show an increase in the T cell population from about 5 hours to a maximum at around 72 hours after solar simulated irradiation; initially CD4+ T cells are seen while later CD8+ T cells and Langerhans cells predominate.

It is known that in normal individuals, UVB exposure induces local immune suppression in the skin; this could be viewed as being advantageous in preventing immune reactions to UV-induced neo-antigens. From this standpoint, it has been postulated that PLE develops where there is a failure in this immunosuppressive mechanism. Kolgen *et al*[6] have demonstrated several differences in the response to UVB exposure between normal controls and PLE patients. Broadly, in PLE patients there was impaired migration Langerhans cells (CD1a+) from the epidermis, which appeared to be related to decreased numbers of cells expressing promigratory cytokines IL-1-β and TNF-α. Migration into the epidermis of CD11b+ cells was marked in normal individuals but sparse in PLE patients despite their substantial numbers in the dermis. Immunohistochemical double staining techniques have shown these cells to be mainly neutrophils (CD11b+ CD68-) in normal subjects as compared with macrophages (CD11b+ CD68+) in PLE subjects; the lack of epidermal neutrophils expressing the immunosuppressive cytokine IL-10 could allow an immune response manifest as PLE to follow UV exposure. Studies of cytokine profiles in UVB-exposed skin in PLE patients have shown fewer cells expressing IL-4, which favors a Th1 response. These factors point to the erythema response in PLE overshadowing the immunosuppressive response to UVB exposure.

Clinical presentation

The condition commonly presents in spring or early summer as a pruritic, erythematous, papular rash on exposed sites. The rash may be preceded by a burning or tingling sensation and usually develops within 30 minutes to several hours of sun exposure; rarely, this latency period extends to 1–3 days. The perennially exposed sites like the hands and face can be spared, with the rash most affecting the sites revealed by summer apparel, such as the neck, forearms, and legs. Frequently, the papules are just 1–2 mm in diameter but can be larger or confluent and thus forming plaques. Several morphologic types have been described: papular, plaque, papulovesicular, vesicobullous, hemorrhagic, and erythema multiforme-like. A form known as PLE sine eruptione describes a sunlight-induced pruritus without a rash. Recently, a pinpoint form has been described in dark skin. A limited form of PLE presenting as a papulovesicular eruption

on the helices of the ears, usually in boys in springtime, is called juvenile spring eruption. The term PLE reflects these different forms, but, for the individual, a particular morphology tends to prevail leading to a mainly monomorphic picture, which is usually consistent between attacks (36-43).

The rash resolves without scarring in about 1–14 days in the absence of further sun exposure. Over the course of the summer, the intensity of the eruption diminishes with further sun exposure. This tolerance is known as "hardening" and probably accounts for the relative sparing of perennially exposed sites. The condition remits over the winter months and persistence of a rash, often of an eczematous or pruriginous nature, should prompt reconsideration of the differential diagnosis. It is of course possible to see PLE provoked by strong winter sunlight, especially in the presence of snow, which results in high levels of reflected light and consequent involvement of shadow sites. Artificial sources emitting some ultraviolet light, such as arc welding equipment and photocopiers, have also been reported to cause PLE.

Differential diagnosis

Subacute cutaneous lupus erythematosus (SCLE) can be provoked by sun exposure and may display similar clinical features. Indeed, there is a high prevalence of PLE in LE patients and their first-degree relatives, suggesting a shared pathogenesis.

Contact dermatitis to sunscreens may cause initial diagnostic difficulty, which can be resolved by patch testing if suspected. Actinic prurigo and PLE can be inseparable in borderline cases, although, over a period of years, clinical progression to one or other may occur. These overlap cases, possibly in an evolving state, have been labeled as persistent polymorphic light eruption (PPLE). Genetic studies suggest that AP may represent a subset of PLE defined by particular human leukocyte antigens.[4]

An uncommon form of solar urticaria in which the rash appears several hours after sun exposure can be mistaken for PLE and indeed solar urticaria has been reported to progress to PLE. The evolution, age of onset, and eventual scarring distinguish hydroa vacciniforme from PLE, as does histologic examination, but the early picture of both can be similar. The cutaneous porphyrias and the photo-aggravated dermatoses such as Jessner's lymphocytic infiltrate are infrequently confused with PLE.

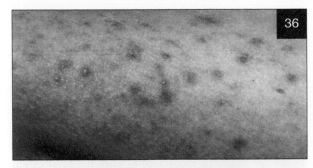

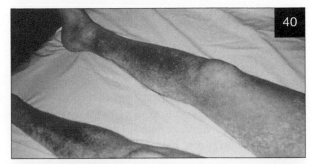

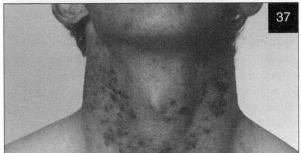

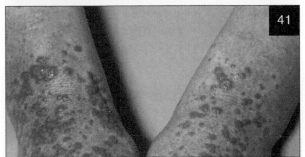

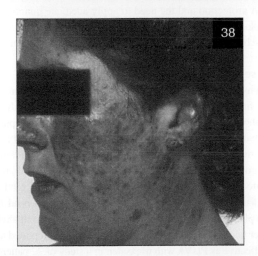

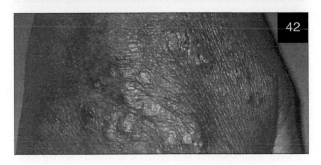

36: Papular PLE.
37: PLE with sparing of shadow sites.
38: Papular and plaque PLE.
39: Impetiginized papulovesicular PLE.

40: Hemorrhagic PLE.
41: EM morphology PLE in acral distribution.
42: Lichenified PLE.
43: PLE affecting pinna.

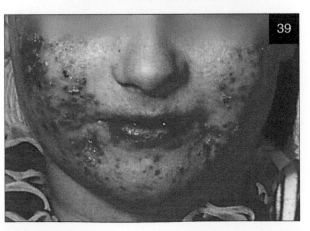

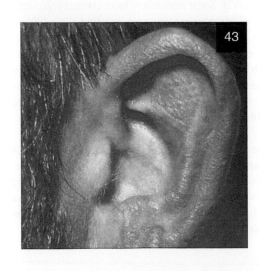

Investigations

The high prevalence of PLE in patients with lupus erythematosus, together with the different and potentially conflicting therapeutic implications, requires that the antinuclear antibody (ANA) and, more specifically, the anti-Ro and La antibody serology should be defined. Screening with plasma spectrofluorimetry or quantitative measurements of urine, stool, and red cell porphyrins should be done if porphyria is being considered.

Histology
There is a wide spectrum of non-specific histologic appearances for PLE, reflecting the varied morphologies and overlap with AP (44).

Phototesting
Monochromator and solar simulator minimal erythema dose testing were shown to be normal in 134 out of 582 patients when testing on the upper back or buttock skin. However, such tests have implicated UVA wavelengths between 320 and 400 nm in two-thirds of PLE patients as being associated with reduced minimal erythema thresholds. Smaller proportions display abnormal sensitivity in the UVB range or across a broadband spanning UVB, UVA, and visible wavelengths. Such testing rarely provokes the morphology of the sun-induced lesions (45, 46).

Provocation tests
PLE lesions can be provoked more reliably using repetitive doses from higher output UV sources than the monochromator or solar simulator. It is best done on normally affected sites, particularly in the winter months when natural photoprotection is at a nadir but even then may be unsuccessful in 10–20% of patients. UVA was found to be more effective in provoking lesions in some studies while others were more successful using UVB. Some researchers have claimed enhanced sensitivity of testing using consecutive UVA1 (340–400 nm) and UVB irradiation. Also, repetitive polychromatic phototesting has been advanced as a prognostic tool for distinguishing a "high likelihood of remission" and chronic subgroups of PLE patients, but confirmatory studies are required. Other observers have suggested that shorter UVA and UVB wavelengths may inhibit longer wavelength induction of PLE (47).

In the context of considering the action spectrum of PLE, it is of interest that there is a higher proportion of UVA to UVB in sunlight reaching temperate versus tropical zones and in spring compared with summer sunlight. This might explain the higher prevalence of PLE in temperate climes in springtime. Conversely, a higher UVB content may exert some inhibitory action.

Management

The majority of sufferers with mild PLE probably never seek medical advice and manage their condition by sun avoidance or the use of a sunscreen. Patients should be advised to avoid the hours of maximal UV exposure between 10am and 4pm, to use photoprotective clothing such as broad-brimmed hats and closely woven fabrics and to apply broad-spectrum sunscreens prior to sun exposure. Gradually increasing exposure to sunlight should be encouraged to allow the development of natural tolerance or "hardening".

Sunscreens
The wide spectrum of wavelengths implicated in provocation of PLE means that high-factor, broad-spectrum sunscreens are required. Those containing physical blocks like titanium dioxide are required to screen UVA efficiently. Protection in the near UVA/visible spectrum carries the cosmetic disadvantage of whiteness, caused by the larger particle sizes of pigment needed. The inadequacy of the SPF alone as a measure of UVA protection and the need to apply adequate quantities of sunblock need to be emphasized. However, even with compliance, these basic measures provide inadequate control in many sufferers.

Desensitization
Prophylactic use of photo(chemo)therapy is also of significant benefit to most patients, especially those more severely affected or those who find sunscreens cosmetically unacceptable; increasingly, narrowband UVB is the first choice for all cases. The method, which mirrors the natural observed "hardening" phenomenon, involves graded exposure to UV light. Photochemotherapy, using a psoralen followed by UVA irradiation (PUVA), is of similar efficacy to narrowband (311 nm) phototherapy using the Phillips TL-01 source[7] and slightly better than broadband UVB. UVA alone has been reported to be as effective as PUVA with trioxsalen in a study of 22 patients.

The regimens used vary but typically involve treatment two or three times per week for 4–6 weeks just prior to the sunshine season. If practical, determine the MED, or the minimum phototoxic dose (MPD) for PUVA, and a starting dose of 50–70% of this value. Thereafter, the dose is increased in 10–20% increments at each exposure depending on the response. Where provocation tests have revealed sensitivity primarily in the UVA, it would seem reasonable to start with narrowband UVB and vice versa for sensitivity confined to the UVB. Such information may not be available and, as many patients display broadband sensitivity, the choice between PUVA and UVB phototherapy is determined by other factors:

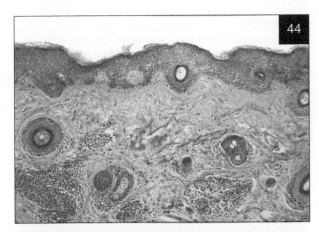

44: Periadnexal lymphohistiocytic infiltrate.
45: PLE provoked in UVA by monochromator phototesting.

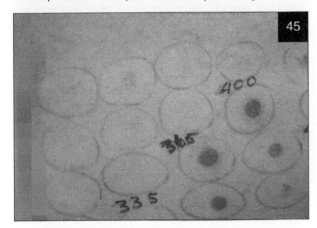

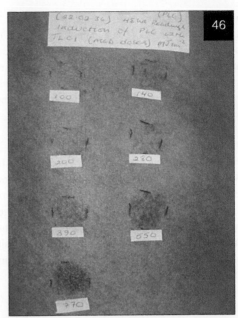

46: PLE provoked by narrowband UVB.

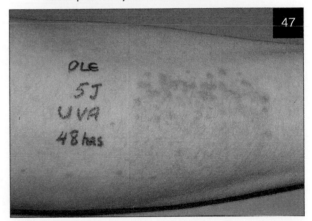

47: Provocation of PLE by 5 J/cm² UVA at 48 hours.

- past responses to treatment
- the avoidance of PUVA in pregnancy
- the need to wear protective sunglasses for 24 hours after oral psoralens
- evidence for carcinogenesis following PUVA, albeit in a psoriasis population.

PLE is commonly provoked during desensitization, occurring in almost half of treatment courses in some series but usually the treatments can be continued with the concomitant use of a moderately potent/potent topical steroid on the affected areas (**48**). After the course is complete, the patient should be advised to maintain their tolerance by continued, careful exposure to sunlight.

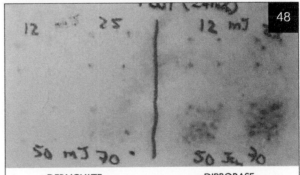

DERMOVATE   DIPROBASE
Positive PLE provocation test at 24h after TL-01 irradiation
Potent topical steroid suppressed the papular response

48: Suppression of PLE by potent topical steroid.

Immunosuppressive therapy

Potent, topical steroids are of value in mild to moderate PLE, as are oral steroids for short periods in settling severe episodes. Low dose azathioprine has been reported as effective in suppressing PLE refractory to other treatments, and cyclosporin used in treating a patient with psoriasis was incidentally noted to reduce the severity of co-existing PLE.

Other drugs

A number of systemic therapies have been tried in the past with little or no proven benefit. These would include chloroquine and quinacrine, thalidomide, beta-carotene, nicotinamide and *Escherichia coli* filtrate (Colibiogen®). A more recent suggestion is that omega-3 polyunsaturated fatty acids in dietary fish oils may decrease the sensitivity to UVA provocation but this is still to be confirmed in clinical practice.

References

1. Pao C, Norris PG, Corbett M et al. Polymorphic light eruption: prevalence in Australia and England. *Br J Dermatol* 1994;**130**:62–4.

2. Frain-Bell W. The idiopathic photodermatoses. In: Frain-Bell W, ed. *Cutaneous Photobiology,* 1st edn. New York: Oxford University Press, 1985.

3. Epstein S. Studies in abnormal human sensitivity to light. IV. Photo-allergic concept of prurigo aestivalis. *J Invest Dermatol* 1942;**5**:289–95.

4. McGregor JM, Grabczynska S, Vaughan R, Hawk JLM, Lewis CM. Genetic modeling of abnormal photosensitivity in families with polymorphic light eruption and actinic prurigo. *J Invest Dermatol* 2000;**115**: 471–6.

5. Norris PG, Hawk JLM, White IR. Photo-allergic contact dermatitis from Fentichlor. *Contact Dermatitis* 1988;**18**:318–20.

6. Kölgen W, van Weelden H, den Hengst et al. CD11b+ cells and ultraviolet-B-resistant CD1a+ cells in skin of patients with polymorphous light eruption. *J Invest Dermatol* 1999;**113**: 4–10.

7. Bilsland D, George S, Gibbs NK, Ferguson J. A comparison of narrowband phototherapy (TL-01) and photochemotherapy (PUVA) in the management of polymorphic light eruption. *Br J Dermatol* 1993;**129**:708–12.

6 Hydroa Vacciniforme
Girish Gupta

Hydroa vacciniforme (HV) is a rare idiopathic photo-dermatosis first described by Bazin in 1862. It is characterized by vesicles and crust formation after sunlight exposure. The lesions typically occur on photo-exposed sites, may persist for several weeks and heal with varioliform scarring. HV usually presents in childhood with spontaneous improvement during adolescence. Parents generally seek specialist advice as their children are unable to tolerate sunshine (play outdoors or travel abroad) and the eruption can result in considerable scarring, leading to significant morbidity.

There have been three case series,[1-3] in addition to a number of case reports, published in the literature.

Epidemiology

Incidence
The true incidence has not been documented. However, the Scottish case review estimated the prevalence to be 1 case per 300,000 population.[3]

Age of onset
HV typically occurs in early childhood and clears spontaneously in adolescence. There are the occasional reports of it occurring in infancy[2] and in the elderly. The mean age of onset has been reported to be between 6 and 8 years.[1,3] More recently a bimodal age distribution has been noted (49), with patients presenting in early childhood (1–7 years) or around/after puberty (12–16 years).[3]

Sex distribution
Both sexes are affected equally,[3] although earlier reports suggested a female preponderance.[2] A recent review suggested that females have an earlier onset (mean 6.7 years) than males (mean 8.7 years) (49). Males also have a longer duration of symptoms than females.[3]

Familial cases
The disease is sporadic. However, there are three reports of HV affecting identical twins and siblings.[1] The reason for this is not known.

Mechanism

The pathogenesis of HV is not clear. Although sensitivity to UVB has been suggested, there is strong evidence that points towards the longer UV wavelengths as the more likely causal factor. The wavelengths implicated vary between 320 and 390 nm,[2,3] with some patients being photosensitive in the visible light spectrum.[3] In addition to reduced UVA MED values,[2] repetitive broad-spectrum UVA has been shown to reproduce lesions that are clinically and histologically identical to those produced by natural sunlight and that heal with scarring.[4]

The chromophore leading to UV-induced damage in HV is unknown. Previous *in vitro* studies with serum lymphocytes and fibroblasts have suggested a reduction in DNA repair following UV exposure. However, these findings remain unconfirmed. Results from pyridoxine toxicity studies have suggested that its photoproducts may be involved in causing tissue damage either directly or via DNA. However, the origin of these molecules remains unknown.

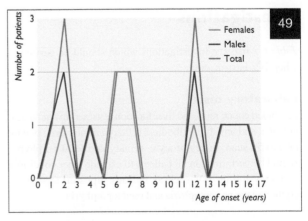

49: Age of onset of HV.

Latent Epstein–Barr virus has been found in the dermal infiltrates of patients with HV. These reports are from South-East Asia, particularly Japan.[5] These findings have not been reported from North America or Europe, nor has active Epstein–Barr virus been documented in this condition. The presence of latent Epstein–Barr virus may reflect the endemic distribution of this in Japan and other South-East Asian countries. The exact role of sunlight and Epstein–Barr virus in HV has yet to be elucidated.

Reports of familial cases of HV raise the possibility of genetic determinants underlying susceptibility to this condition. Tissue typing in patients with HV has shown a significant association with HLA DR4 and HLA DR53 (G Gupta, unpublished observations, 2002) but the mechanism of cell damage has not been determined.

Clinical presentation

The onset of the eruption is usually seasonal, in the spring or summer, although some patients have symptoms throughout the year. After exposure to sunlight, itchy tender papules and vesicles appear on a background of edematous erythema, primarily on photo-exposed sites (50). This is followed by a phase of impetiginized or hemorrhagic crusting (51, 52), and the lesions eventually heal with characteristic vario-liform scarring (53). The sites most commonly involved include the cheeks, ears, nose, and dorsa of the hands.
Uncommon presentations of HV include eye involvement, such as conjunctival injection, herpes keratitis, photophobia, corneal ulceration, and scarring. Other rare features include deformities of the ear and nose and contractures of the fingers.[4]

Investigations

Table 6.1 lists the investigations which should be performed when HV is suspected.

Laboratory tests

Full blood count; renal and liver function tests; serum antinuclear, anti-Ro, and anti-La antibodies; urinary amino acids; plasma porphyrin scan; or erythrocyte, urinary and fecal porphyrins should be performed in all patients to exclude other conditions that may mimic HV such as bullous lupus erythematosus, erythropoietic protoporphyria and pseudoporphyria.

Narrowband UVB (TL-01) minimal erythema dose (MED)

In general, this is normal in patients with HV.

Monochromator tests

These essentially demonstrate photosensitivity in the UVA spectrum.

UVA provocation tests

These may be difficult to perform on particularly young children. However, they show changes and result in scarring, similar to that seen in patients with HV triggered by sunshine (54).

Histology

Spongiosis is seen in the early stages of HV, which may be in the form of an intraepidermal spongiotic vesicle, or it may become more widespread in cases of severe disease. A diffuse upper dermal lymphocytic infiltrate and areas of keratinocyte necrosis are also seen (see Chapter 15).

Management

This is summarized in Table 6.2. Due to the rare nature of this condition, there are no large, randomized trials in the literature. Evidence for treatment comes from case series and single reports.[6]

First-line therapy

Patients should initially receive treatment with high-factor broad-spectrum sunscreens and advice on behavioral sunlight avoidance. Windows in the car and home should be covered with Dermaguard Film (manufactured by Sun Guard, Florida, USA), which prevents the penetration of UV

Table 6.1: Investigations in hydroa vacciniforme

Laboratory
Full blood count
Renal function tests
Liver function tests
Antinuclear antibody
Anti-Ro and anti-La antibodies
Urinary amino acids
Plasma porphyrin scan
or
Erythrocyte, urinary and fecal porphyrins
Phototesting
Narrowband UVB (TL-01) MED
Monochromator tests
UVA provocation tests
Skin biopsy

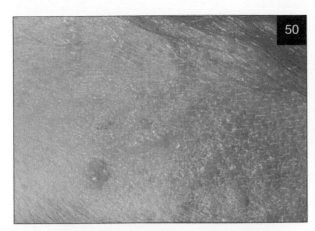

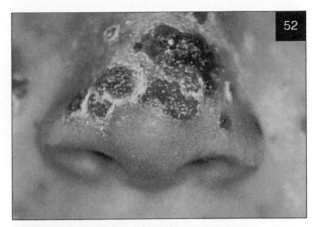

50: Early clinical features showing vesicles on a photo-exposed site.
51: Hemorrhagic crusts seen on the ear.

52: Hemorrhagic crusts and necrosis seen on the nose.
53: Varioliform scarring as end result of tissue damage.

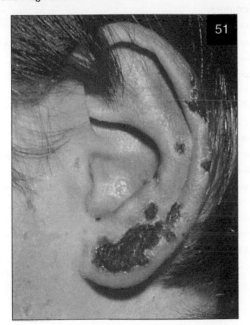

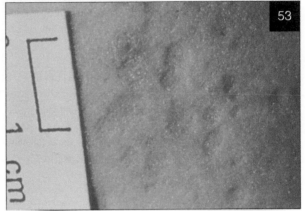

Table 6.2: Management of hydroa vaccinlforme

First-line therapy
High-factor broad-spectrum sunscreens
Behavioral sunlight avoidance
DermaGard Film

Second-line therapy
Narrowband UVB (TL-01) phototherapy

Third-line therapy
Hydroxychloroquine, chloroquine
Beta-carotene
Dietary fish oils
PUVA
Azathioprine
Ciclosporin

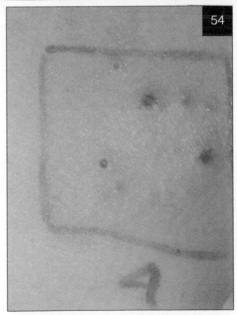

54: HV-like lesions induced by UVA following UVA photoprovocation tests.

wavelengths <380 nm. This conservative approach is satisfactory in the majority of patients.[3]

Second-line therapy

Narrowband UVB (TL-01) phototherapy has been used to successfully treat those patients who continue to develop new lesions despite these conservative measures. Treatment is generally given 10 times in early spring to prevent the summer flare.[3,7] Should this approach fail, then alternative treatments should be sought.

Third-line therapy

The use of antimalarials has been reported with variable results. Hydroxychloroquine 100 mg daily seems to be ineffective, but at higher doses of 200 mg daily or b.i.d. it may result in disease improvement in a few patients. Chloroquine sulfate 100–125 mg daily has also been shown to decrease the severity of disease.[2] Chloroquine phosphate 500 mg daily and mepacrine were ineffective.

Traditionally, beta-carotene has been used when conservative measures have failed, probably due to a low incidence of toxicity. Results are variable with only a few reports suggesting that beta-carotene 180 mg daily decreased the severity of disease. The majority of studies, however, show that beta-carotene 100–200 mg daily was ineffective.

In one report, dietary fish oil rich in omega-3 polyunsaturated fatty acids, five capsules daily for 3 months, was given to three patients, with clinical improvement noted in two of them. The mechanism may be through inhibition of prostanoid production and by its proposed buffering effect against free radical-induced damage.

PUVA has been used in five patients in separate reports, being ineffective in three cases. In the other two cases, it was reported to be helpful but, in one of these cases, the patient was also on prednisolone 40 mg daily with initial improvement but no long-lasting remission.

For severe and refractory HV unresponsive to other therapies, immunosuppressive agents including azathioprine and ciclosporin may be effective but thalidomide does not seem to be.

References

1. McGrae J D Jr, Perry HO. Hydroa vacciniforme. *Arch Dermatol* 1963;**87**:618–25.
2. Sonnex TS, Hawk JLM. Hydroa vacciniforme: a review of ten cases. *Br J Dermatol* 1988;**118**:101–8.
3. Gupta G, Man I, Kemmett D. Hydroa vacciniforme: a clinical and follow-up study of 17 cases. *J Am Acad Dermatol* 2000;**42**:208–13.
4. Hann S K, Im S, Park Y-K, Lee S. Hydroa vacciniforme with unusually severe scar formation: diagnosis by repetitive UVA phototesting. *J Am Acad Dermatol* 1991;**25**:401–3.
5. Iwatsuki K, Xu Z, Takata M et al. Association of latent Epstein–Barr virus infection with hydroa vacciniforme. *Br J Dermatol* 1998;**140**:715–21.
6. Gupta G. Hydroa vacciniforme. In: Lebwohl M, Heymann W, Berth-Jones J, Coulson I, eds. *Treatment of Skin Disease*, 1st edn. London, Mosby, 2002.
7. Collins P, Ferguson J. Narrow-band UVB (TL-01) phototherapy: an effective preventative treatment for the photodermatoses. *Br J Dermatol* 1995;**132**:956–63.

7 Chronic Actinic Dermatitis

James Ferguson

Chronic actinic dermatitis (CAD), which is a term synonymous with the photosensitivity dermatitis and actinic reticuloid (PD/AR) syndrome, is a member of the idiopathic photodermatoses. This condition, which is not rare, can in its severe form be extremely disabling, leading to a nocturnal existence and even suicide. All patients have abnormal photosensitivity to ultraviolet and, in 50%, visible wavelengths. The majority also have multiple contact allergies, which in about half precede the development of photosensitivity. The clinical presentation ranges from a dermatitis reaction with, on occasions, depigmentation to a pseudolymphomatous actinic reticuloid skin state. Many patients have covered site involvement and may even present with erythroderma. Phototesting and patch testing are the key investigations. Photopatch testing, which is frequently difficult because of a positive UVA irradiation control reaction, unfortunately rarely provides useful additional information.

Mechanism

The cause(s) of CAD remains unknown. On current evidence, it seems likely that there is a subtle immunologic abnormality that results in hypersensitivity to UV/visible wavelength altered skin elements. In a similar fashion, multiple contact allergy, again presumably due to either loss of tolerance or an exaggerated allergic response to agents with which we are all in common contact, suddenly produces a significant clinical problem. It seems likely that the mechanism for this is likely to be a T lymphocyte-mediated delayed-type hypersensitivity with loss of normal modulation. It is true, however, that we are unable to pinpoint the precise cause and, indeed, in those patients who spontaneously improve, the reason why this condition can resolve is unknown.

Epidemiology

Incidence

CAD is one of the most frequently encountered photodermatoses in patients >50 years of age. It is characterized by a dermatitis reaction, which may with chronic light or contact allergen stimulation enter a pseudolymphomatous state.

The precise incidence is unknown. Within the Tayside region of Scotland (population 500,000) approximately 1:6000 will develop CAD. The ratio of male to female is 9:1 and as yet there is no clear evidence that a particular type of employment (outdoor or indoor) or exposure to chemicals related to work or a hobby is associated. It can affect all races, although most of the patients reported are Caucasian.

Clinical presentation

While one might expect all sufferers to present with a clear history of sunlight-induced dermatitis episodes, maximal during the summer sunshine season, this frequently is not the case with a perennial problem reported by most. Many patients have a long history, usually of recurrent multiple contact allergy to initially undefined allergens. In such cases, contact site involvement is usually followed by a perennial exposed site dermatitis, often developing years later. Even at that time, it may be unclear that the exposed site involvement is due to sunlight, presumably because of the varied combination of contact allergies and broad-spectrum ultraviolet and visible photosensitivity. When combined, such factors produce a range of features with most patients showing the clinical and histologic features of a dermatitis (see Chapter 15) involving photo-exposed skin sites of face, neck, ears and backs of hands (55, 56). In others, rarely (<10%), the morphology is of a pseudolymphoma (actinic reticuloid) (57). The sites of photosensitivity involvement are often helpful, as are cut-off lines (58) pointing to the photo-protective position of clothing, sparing beneath the spectacle frames (55), within the hair-bearing scalp areas and behind the ears (59), which are all characteristic features that help alert the clinician to the diagnosis.

On occasions, the presentation can be a generalized erythro-derma with about half of all patients having clothing-covered site involvement at some point in their illness. Others present with contact allergic dermatitis (60) (involvement of eyelids, beneath the chin, and within the ears and hair-bearing scalp), pointing towards contact allergy, which can either be direct contact or airborne; the causal agents must be identified by multiple patch testing to enable avoidance advice.

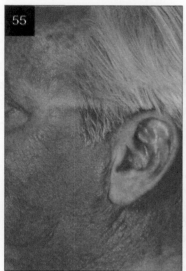

55: A photo-exposed site dermatitis. Note the relative sparing in areas photoprotected by his spectacles and freedom of collar protected skin.

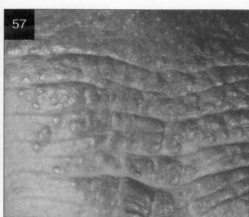

57: Pseudolymphomatous semitranslucent nodules occurring particularly with relative sparing in skin creases (actinic reticuloid).

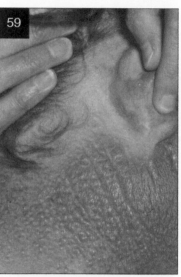

59: Sparing behind the ear in this patient who has pseudolymphomatous nodules (actinic reticuloid) strongly suggesting the main provoking factor in this patient is light.

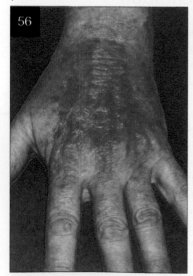

56: A dermatitis response predominantly affecting back of hand with relative sparing of his arm/wrist and fingers.

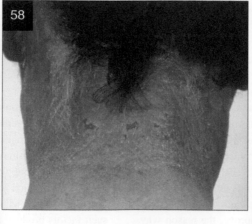

58: An unusually sharp cut-off at the back of this patient's neck demonstrates the photoprotection provided by clothing.

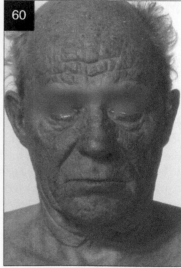

60: Airborne contact allergic ermatitis/ presentation of CAD. Note the eyelid/ infranasal sites are affected.

Investigations

Histopathology of affected skin (see Chapter 15)

At the mild end of the spectrum, the histology is a dermatitis. When chronic stimulation by light or contact allergens occurs, a pseudolymphoma with characteristic atypical lymphocytes having Sezary-like features is seen (actinic reticuloid).

Phototesting

Monochromator wavelength dependency studies of uninvolved mid-upper back skin, avoiding the paravertebral groove area, demonstrate that the whole skin is abnormally sensitive to broad UVB/UVA (**61**) and frequently extends into the visible region (**62**). Although the UVB region is the area of greatest abnormality, the longer wavelengths can be particularly troublesome due to their ability to penetrate clothing and window glass. The phototest morphology is a dermatitis response (**63, 64**) which is valuable both for clinical confirmation of the diagnosis and for investigative study. Repeat phototesting over a period of years allows monitoring of the disease state. It should be noted that some CAD patients who have clinically improved and tolerate sunlight exposure may still have abnormal phototesting on back skin, which raises the possibility of an exposed site desensitization process.

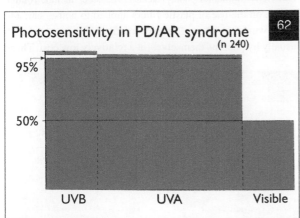

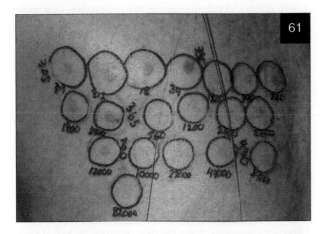

Photosensitivity in PD/AR syndrome (n 240)

95%

50%

UVB   UVA   Visible

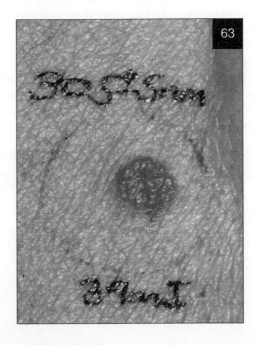

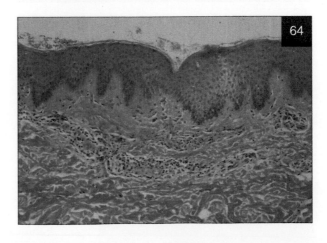

61: Monochromator phototesting demonstrating marked abnormal results typical of chronic actinic dermatitis.

62: The majority of patients demonstrate UVB and A photosensitivity combined; 50% also show extension into the visible region.

63: This UVB 305 ≥ 5 nm phototest site shows an indurated microvesicular response typical of dermatitis and quite different from acute sunburn.

64: This histology of a phototest site demonstrates an acute dermatitis reaction.

Patch testing

Standard patch testing should be conducted to a wide range of test series. Although contact allergy to members of the European Standards series, Compositae and sunscreens has been recorded, other series should be used as required. The majority of patients demonstrate multiple contact allergy (**65**).

Photopatch testing is a difficult investigation when UVA sensitivity is profound. Recently 5 J/cm² of UVA has been routinely used for all patients suspected of photocontact allergy. If the minimal erythemal dose (MED) for an individual CAD patient falls below this level, the presence of a positive irradiation control makes interpretation of results unviable. Lower UVA doses can be used, although eventually they may get below the threshold to trigger the individual's photo-allergy, producing a false-negative result.

Phototest and patch test investigations are sometimes only possible after inpatient treatment in a photoprotective cubicle. Potent topical steroid use does need to be withdrawn (probably for 1 week) before testing to minimize the risk of false-negative results (**66**).

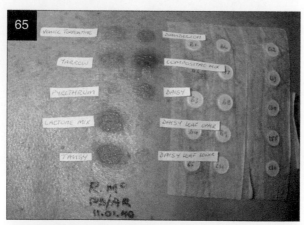

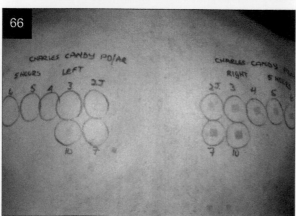

Management

The management of chronic actinic dermatitis requires a firm clinical diagnosis with education about the condition, provision of a patient information sheet, advice on sunlight and allergen avoidance measures and application of appropriate topical therapies.

The information required for each patient should be individualized according to the specific profile of contact allergens and photosensitivity. General information about CAD should be provided for each patient. Written information (available through www.dundee.ac.uk/dermatology/photo/clinical/pdar.html) is an example of what is used in Dundee, and does help newly diagnosed patients take in the information in a more measured fashion than is achieved by a single consultation.

For all patients, sunlight avoidance should be discussed as:
- behavioral measures
- clothing protection
- environmental photoprotection, and
- topical broad-spectrum sunscreens.

All patients should be advised to avoid intense mid-day sunlight (10am–3pm) and to limit outdoor activities to outside these hours. Advice on clothing includes keeping covered up as much as possible, wearing close, tightly woven material, when possible dark colored, to prevent visible wavelength penetration. Other environmental photoprotection measures include routine advice on the use of plastic filters applied to house, car, and work windows. Clear Dermaguard film (**67**) can be fitted, usually by patients themselves, at a relatively low cost. Those

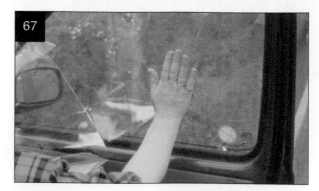

65: Multiple contact allergy is a common finding in CAD. A broad range of agents, including Compositae, are found to be responsible.
66: The left-hand side of this patient's back has been pretreated with Diprosone Ointment while the right hand side was treated with Diprobase Ointment. The influence of steroid in this mirror image phototesting can clearly be seen.
67: Dermaguard photoprotective film can be used at home or in the car.

with visible wavelength sensitivity may consider fitting an orange film, such as Bex Film U (Summerside Blinds, Leith, UK) to house or work windows. This colored film is not legal for car windshields as it may prevent traffic light vision.

Although topical sunscreens are useful, there are problems with insufficient application, which can have a drastic effect on the achieved protection factor. For those patients with a marked visible wavelength sensitivity, a specifically formulated zinc oxide/titanium dioxide can be recommended.[1]

Allergen avoidance is given as written on the contact clinic advice sheets, which are an important method of reinforcing the information. Patch testing is usually repeated every 2 years or so for the range of allergies, as it is an evolving process, particularly with regard to topical therapeutic agents and sunscreens.

Most patients manage with emollients, topical steroids, antigen and photoprotective measures. A minority require desensitization with PUVA or UVB phototherapy. This, however, is not a simple procedure as many are severely photosensitive and fail to tolerate therapy. Others require third-line therapy with cyclosporin or prednisolone.

Some patients find even simple modification of their environment and avoidance of allergens extremely difficult, particularly if they are keen gardeners. Such cases do require more intensive support, often from their spouse.

Prognosis

Although there have been a number of reports of the development of systemic lymphoma, a follow-up study of cancer registry linkage showed no association beyond what would be expected as a chance finding.[2] This study assessed a group of CAD patients managed largely by sunlight and allergen avoidance. It is true that patients with CAD managed with systemic immunosuppressants might be expected to be at a true increased risk.

Some patients do show spontaneous improvement with normalization of phototesting; interestingly, abnormal contact allergies often persist for many years. The probability of a cure, confirmed by normal phototesting, is relatively low with only approximately 20% completely resolving by 10 years after initial diagnosis. CAD patients are, however, pleased to learn that resolution can always occur however long they may have had the condition.[3]

Chronic actinic dermatitis in young atopic dermatitis patients

In 1998, a new group of CAD was identified, which differs significantly from the elderly male-dominated CAD group.[4] These patients who are in their teens and 20s have a childhood history of atopic dermatitis that becomes marked on photo-exposed sites (**68**). While this type was previously considered to be photo-aggravated atopic dermatitis, phototesting and patch testing have revealed the hallmarks of chronic actinic dermatitis–multiple contact allergies and broad-spectrum photosensitivity. These young "outgoing" patients often find it more difficult to avoid ultraviolet and their contact allergens. As a consequence, more seem to require third-line immunosuppressive therapy than the older CAD group. Spontaneous resolution is also reported,[4] even in those who have severe phototest evidence of photosensitivity.

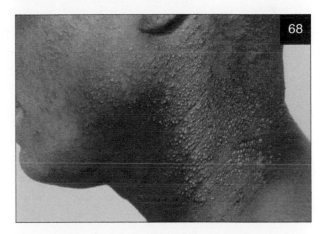

68: A young atopic dermatitis patient with marked photosensitivity affecting his neck.

References

1. Moseley H, Cameron H, MacLeod T, Clark C, Dawe R, Ferguson J. New sunscreens confer improved protection for photosensitive patients in the blue light region. *J Dermatol* 2001;**145**:789–94.

2. Bilsland D, Crombie IK, Ferguson J. The photosensitivity dermatitis and actinic reticuloid syndrome (PD/AR): no association with lymphoreticular malignancy. *Br J Dermatol* 1994;**131**:209–14.

3. Dawe RS, Crombie IK, Ferguson J. The natural history of chronic actinic dermatitis. *Arch Dermatol* 2000;**136**:1215–20.

4. Russell SC, Dawe RS, Collins P, Man I, Ferguson J. The photosensitivity dermatitis and actinic reticuloid syndrome (chronic actinic dermatitis) occurring in seven young atopic dermatitis patients. *Br J Dermatol* 2000;**138**:496–501.

5. Schuster C, Zepter K, Kempf W, Dummer R. Successful treatment of recalcitrant chronic acitnic dermatitis with tacrilimus. *Dermatology* 2004;**209**:325-328.

8 Solar Urticaria
Paula Beattie

Solar urticaria (SU) is an uncommon photodermatosis, which is an immediate-type hypersensitivity reaction, usually to UVA (320–400 nm) and visible (400–700 nm), less often to UVB (290–320 nm) and rarely to infrared radiation. It is characterized by itching, erythema, and whealing over sun-exposed sites, which, when severe, cause significant lifestyle restriction. It is usually idiopathic but can be seen in association with porphyria, drugs, and topical tar.

Epidemiology

Onset can be at any age, with a peak incidence between the third and fifth decades. It accounts for less than 1% of cases of urticaria. Prevalence in the Tayside region of Scotland is estimated to be 3.1 per 100,000 of the population with 70% female predominance, but no variation in incidence with skin type.[1] SU can be seen in conjunction with chronic idiopathic and other physical urticarias as well as with other photodermatoses such as polymorphic light eruption and chronic actinic dermatitis.

Mechanism

SU represents an immediate type I hypersensitivity, antigen–antibody reaction to radiation. The activating wavelengths convert a chromophore (pro-antigen) into an antigen by photochemical alteration. This is recognized by specific IgE to this allergen on the surface of mast cells, causing degranulation and release of histamine and other mediators.[2] These mediators increase vascular permeability, which allows dermal leakage of fluid, causing a wheal (69).

In the fixed form, mast cell alteration within a localized area is proposed. When solar urticaria is caused by drug ingestion, it is felt that the drug or its metabolites act as a chromophore. When seen in association with porphyria, the porphyrins are the chromophore. A classification of different types of SU was proposed according to the action spectra and immunologic factors. However, action spectra can vary over time in an individual patient and the pathogenesis would appear to be more complex than this classification allows for.

Clinical presentation

There is a wide variety in both the spectrum of clinical disease and the wavelengths responsible in individual patients. The onset of SU is frequently sudden and can be clearly recalled by the majority of patients. It is characterized by itch and/or a burning sensation, then erythema and usually, but not always, whealing over sun-exposed sites. Most commonly this includes the "V" of neck and arms, with less severe involvement of the more habitually exposed face and hands, which develop natural "hardening". An uncommon form, fixed SU, affects only localized areas of skin and will recur in these sites on re-exposure.

Urticaria develops after only seconds of sun exposure in the most severely affected but after 5 minutes of exposure in approximately 50% and after 15 minutes in another 25%. In a few, long exposure times of an hour or more are necessary to provoke urticaria and can lead to confusion with immediate - onset polymorphic light eruption, so that phototesting is necessary to provide a definitive diagnosis. Severity and therefore exposure time necessary for provocation can vary in any one patient over time and be affected by season, altitude, latitude, and reflection. The short exposure times required in the majority of patients mean that this disease has major lifestyle implications, many being almost housebound prior

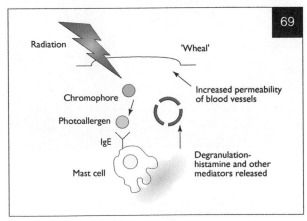

69: Solar urticaria to a number of wavelengths.

to diagnosis and treatment. The latent period between sun exposure and onset of signs or symptoms will usually be <2 hours but rarely can be more prolonged (delayed-onset solar urticaria), again possibly leading to confusion with polymorphic light eruption.

SU lesions persist for <2 hours in around 60% and up to 24 hours in the rest. In those who also suffer from polymorphic light eruption, a papular rash supersedes the urticaria and persists for much longer periods.

Around 80% of patients report urticaria provocation through thin clothing. They will, however, be protected by thicker or more than one layer of clothing and exhibit sparing beneath underwear or the cuffs/collars of shirts (**70**), and under jewelry (**71**) and footwear (**72**). Different types and colors of fabric allow variable transmission of radiation (**72**). The majority of patients are sensitive to UVA and visible wavelengths, which can pass through window or windscreen glass (**70**). They experience perennial SU, as both UVA and visible radiation show little seasonal variation.

Other sources of radiation capable of provoking solar urticaria include UVA sun beds and indoor lighting. Intense exposure of large areas of skin, such as occurs while a sun bed is being used, can lead to systemic symptoms including dizziness, nausea, and potentially fatal hypotension.

Histopathology

SU is associated with a vascular and perivascular infiltrate of neutrophils and eosinophils (mast cells) in lesional skin within minutes of irradiation followed by a gradual increase in cell numbers as a result of recruitment by released chemotactic factors (cytokines) from degranulated mast cells (see Chapter 15). These cytokines may contribute to the endothelial swelling of dermal vessels and resulting fluid leakage, manifest as upper dermal spongiosis.

Action spectrum

Most commonly UVA (320–400 nm) and visible (400–600 nm) wavelengths are responsible for solar urticaria with a small proportion of patients also sensitive to UVB (290–320 nm), and a smaller number again to infrared wavelengths. Patients may have SU provoked by only a single waveband, but the majority will demonstrate sensitivity to many (**73**). If SU is seen at only 430/460 ± 30 nm (**74**), SU secondary to porphyria or a drug should be considered. A number of patients have "inhibition spectra" whereby simultaneous or immediate post-irradiation with wavelengths longer (less often shorter) than those eliciting urticaria will inhibit the response.[3]

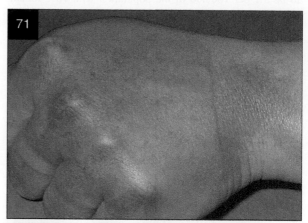

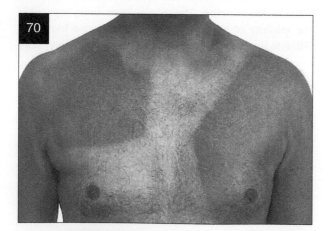

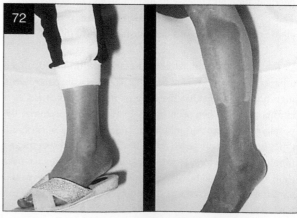

70: Patient affected through a car window, exhibiting sparing under collar, lapels and seat belt.
71: Swelling of the hand with sparing under the ring which has been removed.
72: Solar urticaria provoked through the lighter but not the darker fabric and sparing under the patients footwear.

Chromophores

Chromophores are molecules capable of absorbing specific wavelengths of radiation. Some cutaneous chromophores responsible for solar urticaria can also be detected in the serum of some patients. In these it is possible to passively transfer solar urticaria to a non-affected individual by intradermal injection of their serum (passive transfer test). For ethical reasons this is no longer carried out as it carries a risk of transferring blood borne disease.

Patients with a photo-allergen present in the serum will react to intradermal injection of their own plasma after it has been irradiated *in vitro* (intradermal test) (75). In such cases, and in some with negative intradermal tests, plasma exchange therapy can provide therapeutic benefit by removal of the circulating plasma factor.

A circulating allergen has been demonstrated in the serum of some patients but not chemically identified. In view of the heterogeneity of action spectra seen in different patients, it would appear reasonable to assume that a range of chromophores are responsible.

Mediators

Histamine is important in about two-thirds of patients who have complete good, or partial response to antihistamines. A rise in plasma histamine in the venous blood draining irradiated sites can be found, and there may be an increase in numbers of histamine-releasing mast cells in the skin of SU wheals. Depleting histamine by repeated injection of a mast cell degranulator, then irradiating the same area of skin, can abolish the urticarial response. However, antihistamines will reduce whealing but not flare and therefore other mediators must play a role. Those proposed include acetylcholine, serotonin, kinins, and substance P. Increased numbers of eosinophils are found in urticarial wheals and these secrete leukotriene C4 and platelet-activating factor, which may be involved in wheal production.

Tolerance

The mechanism of UV or visible light-induced tolerance is not fully understood. Those with severe SU are rarely able to expose their skin for long enough to build up tolerance. But, for those milder cases, repeated skin exposure to natural sunlight can lead to a natural "hardening" so that a longer period or more intense exposure is necessary to provoke urticaria. In these patients, lesions will be provoked more easily on the "V" of neck and arms with relative sparing of the more habitually exposed face and hands. Proposed mechanisms include saturation of IgE binding sites, alteration of the photo-allergen or chromophore in the skin or UV-induced

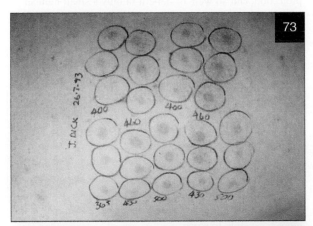

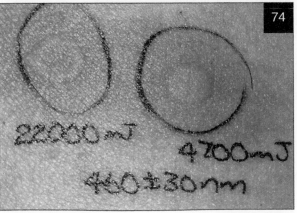

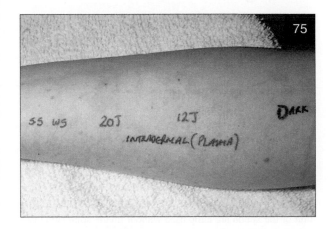

73: Urticarial wheal formation.
74: Solar urticaria at only 430 or 460 nm should raise the suspicion of porphyria or drug etiology.
75: Intradermal test.

suppression of the immune system, by for example depletion of mast cells or degranulation of the mast cells. Thickening or tanning of the epidermis, so that solar radiation to the dermal mast cells is reduced, may also contribute. This phenomenon can be exploited for treatment of SU with incremental exposure to artificial light sources inducing tolerance to natural sunlight.

Differential diagnosis

Other conditions that can give rise to urticaria on exposure to sunlight (*Table 8.1*) include heat urticaria in response to radiant heat from the sun's rays, which can present with a similar history and in a few patients co-exists. These patients may describe the occurrence of urticaria after exposure to artificial sources of heat such as kitchen appliances or a hot shower, and may not describe urticaria on cool sunny days. Heat urticaria can also be provoked during phototesting as a result of heat from the light source at high intensities and so response to an artificial source of infrared radiation or a hot test tube is necessary to exclude this.

As patients with porphyria can develop SU as a feature of their disease, all should have plasma porphyrin screening. Patients should also have serology to exclude lupus.

A number of drugs have been reported to cause SU and a detailed drug history should be elicited. These include NSAIDs, tetracyclines, chlorpromazine and reprinast.

Investigations

Serum
All patients should have a plasma porphyrin screen, autoantibodies and routine hematologic and biochemical parameters.

Monochromator phototesting
To establish the diagnosis and wavelengths dependency, monochromator phototesting is a useful investigation. In centers where such testing is unavailable, this can be carried out using a modified slide projector as a visible source and UVB and UVA phototherapy units. In a few, provocation of urticaria may require irradiation with multiple wavelengths such as are delivered from a broadband UVA or UVB phototherapy unit or the xenon arc lamp used without filters (solar simulated radiation [SSR]), which delivers all wavebands simultaneously. If these measures fail, natural sunlight can be used in an attempt to provoke urticaria before the diagnosis is excluded.

Knowledge of a patient's action spectrum enables advice on light avoidance measures, choice of sunscreen and the phototherapy that would be most suitable for that patient. Assessment of the minimal dose required to provoke urticaria in mJ or J/cm^2 at each affected wavelength, the minimal urticaria dose (MUD), can be used to determine clinical severity, monitor for improvement, and as an objective measure of response to antihistamines or other therapies (**76**).

Management

Sunlight avoidance
As with all photosensitive patients, appropriate sunlight avoidance measures and use of UV protective clothing and broad-brimmed hats should be advised (**77**). For those who are UVA wavelength sensitive, a clear film (museum film) that allows transmission of only small amounts of UVA radiation can be applied to the inside of domestic and car windows.

Sunscreens
In the past, sunscreens have provided UVB but little UVA protection, and so were of benefit in only a small number of solar urticaria patients. With the introduction of broad-spectrum sunscreens, which provide better UVB and UVA coverage, most patients now feel that they obtain useful benefit.[1] However, the majority of patients with solar urticaria are also visible wavelength sensitive and so will achieve only partial benefit from these sunscreens. They can obtain additional benefit from a sunscreen providing visible wavelength protection (Dundee sunscrean produced at Tayside Pharmaceuticals, Ninewells Hospital, Dundee), but unfortunately the drawback of both broad-spectrum and Dundee sunscreens is a whitish appearance given to the skin caused by reflective particles in the cream, and this reduces compliance. The addition of pigment to the Dundee sunscreen makes this more acceptable to some.

Systemic therapy
Antihistamines remain the mainstay of management in the majority of patients. Apart from these, other systemic therapies tried have provided only limited or no therapeutic benefit. These therapies have all been used in the treatment of other urticarias and each is aimed at preventing a different step in the hypersensitivity reaction. Unlike chronic urticaria, the rarity of this condition means that controlled trials would be extremely difficult, but the determination of minimal urticaria dose provides a subjective measure of benefit (**76**).

Antihistamines

Antihistamines provide some symptom control in over 50% of solar urticaria patients with good or complete control in around 30%.[4] The addition of an H_2 antagonist such as cimetidine or ranitidine may provide additional therapeutic benefit in around two-thirds of patients. Therapeutic effect is dose dependent, and often requires a higher dose than necessary for histamine blockade, so that an additional mechanism of action may contribute to therapeutic effect. Non-sedative antihistamines are generally preferred, as sedation will limit patient acceptability and therefore efficacy.

Phototherapy

The choice of phototherapy will depend on the provoking wavelengths. Therapies used include narrowband UVB (TL-01), UVA, and PUVA, and involve exposing the skin to incremental doses of irradiation starting at a dose below that which provokes urticaria (if a light source of the same waveband as that which provokes urticaria is used). Induction of tolerance with one waveband, however, may confer protection against other parts of the UV and visible spectrum. Hence, in a patient without UVB sensitivity, TL-01 therapy can be used to produce tolerance without the risk of provoking urticaria.

In others with broad wavelength sensitivity including UVB, both PUVA and UVA therapy are of benefit, but PUVA appears to provide a more prolonged benefit. Patients with severe sensitivity may have too low an MUD for PUVA therapy to be successful and may require prior treatment with UVA to achieve some tolerance before psoralens can be introduced. An antihistamine prior to each treatment may help patients tolerate phototherapy. Approximately 15 exposures will allow enough hardening for most patients to receive useful benefit by way of increasing the exposure time necessary to provoke their urticaria. Patients are then advised to continue to expose themselves to natural sunlight for limited periods of time to maintain the tolerance induced by phototherapy. The duration of tolerance achieved by phototherapy is highly variable but some patients have benefit for months. As exposure of a large surface area of skin during phototherapy can induce systemic symptoms, only limited areas should be treated (**78**).

Table 8.1: Causes of solar urticaria

Idiopathic	Cutaneous porphyria	Chemical	Drug
	• Porphyria cutanea tarda	• Tar	• Tetracycline
	• Erythropoietic protoporphyria	• Pitch	• Chlorpromazine
			• Reprinast
			• Benoxaprofen (now withdrawn)

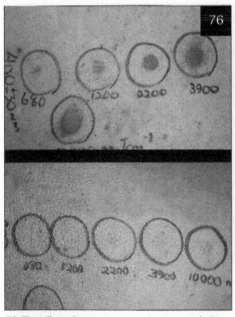

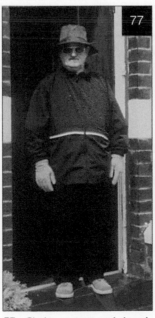

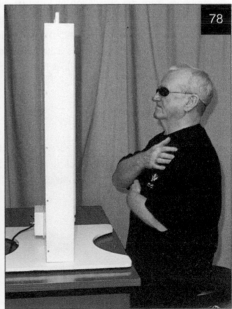

76: The effect of intervention can be measured objectively by assessing the minimal urticaria dose (MUD) before and after.

77: Clothing cover and broad-brimmed hats should be encouraged in addition to sunscreen.

78: Only limited areas should be exposed to prevent provocation of systemic symptoms.

In patients who are visible wavelength sensitive, the wearing of white clothing such as a vest during phototherapy can cause the UVA radiation to be converted to visible wavelengths because of the optical whiteners used during clothing manufacture. This has lead to potentiation of solar urticaria on sites covered by white clothing during phototherapy. In some, sustained hardening is never achieved. In these cases phototherapy can be continued at home with a portable source, the patient receiving daily short exposures.

Other systemic therapy

Those who do not achieve satisfactory symptom control from the above measures may require a trial of other systemic therapies, although response is more often than not disappointing.

- Sodium cromoglycate, nifedipine and ketotifen act by stabilizing the mast cell membrane and therefore degranulation and histamine release but give disappointing results.
- The new leukotriene antagonists, which block leukotriene B4, an inflammatory mediator involved in many allergic responses including asthma and eczema, may potentially help.
- Hydroxychloroquine has been found to benefit a few patients, but beta-carotene and indomethacin are generally unhelpful.
- Immunosuppressive therapies such as corticosteroids and cyclosporin do not help consistently. Intravenous immunoglobulin may help some patients.
- Plasmapheresis (**79**) acts by removing the circulating chromophore from the circulation and can be used in patients with both positive, but also to a lesser degree negative, intradermal plasma tests. Duration of remission is variable, ranging from weeks to years. It is, however, costly, available only in specialist centers and does have associated risks.

Prognosis

SU is a chronic condition. In one series of 57 patients, 22.5%, 57.5% and 73.5% had resolved clinically at 4, 5, and 6 years from onset, respectively.[5] In contrast, we followed up 60

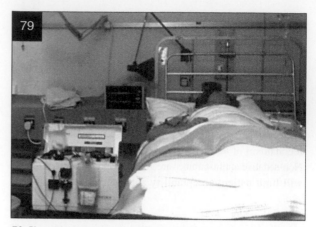

79: Plasmapheresis in a solar urticaria patient.

patients and estimated that at 5, 10, and 15 years from diagnosis, 12%, 26%, and 36% respectively resolved clinically. Repeat phototesting had been carried out in 25 of the 60 patients, and of these, the probability of complete resolution at 5 years was 30%.[1] Age at diagnosis, phototest evidence of severity, wavelengths affected or breadth of action spectrum did not predict outcome. There was a suggestion that the presence of another photodermatosis and older age of diagnosis may result in a worse prognosis.

References

1. Beattie PE, Dawe RS, Ibbotson SH, Ferguson J. The characteristics and prognosis of idiopathic solar urticaria: a cohort of 87 cases. *Arch Dermatol* 2003;**139**:1149–54.

2. Hawk JLM, Eady RAJ, Challoner AVJ, Kobza-Black A, Keahey TM, Greaves MW. Elevated blood histamine levels and mast cell degranulation in solar urticaria. *Br J Clin Pharmacol* 1980;**9**:183–6.

3. Kojima M, Horiko T, Nakamura Y et al. Solar urticaria: relationship of photo-allergen and action spectrum. *Arch Dermatol* 1986;**122**:550–5.

4. Ferguson J. Idiopathic solar urticaria: a natural history and response to non-sedative antihistamine therapy. A study of 26 cases. *Br J Dermatol* 1988;**119**(S33):16.

5. Monfrecola G, Masdturzo E, Riccardo AM, Balato F, Ayala F, Di Costanzo MP. Solar urticaria: a report on 57 cases. *Am J Contact Derm* 2000;**11**:89–94.

9 Actinic Prurigo

Irene Man

Actinic prurigo (AP) is an uncommon, acquired, idiopathic photodermatosis that particularly affects American Indians, and less frequently Caucasian and Asian populations. A variety of descriptions have been used in the past, including Hutchinson's summer prurigo and hereditary polymorphic light eruption (PLE). The term actinic prurigo was introduced in 1961 by Lopez Gonzalez.[1] The disorder has previously been considered to be a variant of PLE, but sufficient differences exist for it to be recognized as a distinct disease entity.

Epidemiology

Incidence
Actinic prurigo has a worldwide distribution. It is most common in American Indians. In Mexico, the disease affects 1.5–3.5% of the general population. The occurrence of the disorder is much lower elsewhere. In Canada, the prevalence has been reported to be 0.1%, and 4% of patients with photodermatoses in a Singapore skin referral center. AP has been reported in Japan, South-East Asia, Europe, and Australia. Familial occurrence is common, with 75–100% reported in American Indians and 50% in Britain.

Age of onset
AP usually manifests in childhood, with the usual age of onset before 10 years. Spontaneous improvement occurs from puberty onwards, with resolution by early adult life in some patients. It has been reported that 62% of these early-onset individuals clear or improve 5 years after initial diagnosis and, in those patients with persistent disease, the disorder tends to be milder in adulthood. There is a subset of patients, especially American Indians (19–28%), who develop symptoms beyond the age of 20 years and, in this group, the disorder tends to be less severe but runs a more chronic course (only 17% reported improvement 5 years after diagnosis).

Sex distribution
AP predominantly affects females, with a female-to-male ratio of 2:1 to 4:1.

Mechanism

The mechanism of AP is unknown. A causal role for UV irradiation is suggested by deterioration of symptoms in summer and abnormal photosensitivity detected on monochromator phototesting in two-thirds of cases. The chromophore involved is unknown. Enhancement of UVB and UVA erythema in the presence of topical indomethacin has been reported, although not confirmed; this may suggest that arachidonic acid metabolism and lipoxygenase derivatives are involved in the pathogenesis of photosensitivity in AP.

Major histocompatibility antigen studies of AP patients have shown a significant positive association with human leukocyte antigens (HLA) A24 and Cw4 in American Indians and with HLA C4 in Colombian patients. A strong association between HLA DR4 (96–100%) and, in particular, the subtype DRB1*0407 (60–72%) has been demonstrated in British Caucasian patients with AP.[2-4] This specific HLA subtype is rare in the general population. Similarly, HLA DR4 has been shown to be present in 93% of Mexican and 86% of Australian AP patients. As with the British Caucasian AP sufferers, a high frequency of the DRB1*0407 allele was detected in these patients. It has been suggested that the presence of this HLA type may have a role in AP disease expression by determining the cutaneous response to a peptide antigen, probably induced by UV radiation, to initiate the clinical manifestations of this disorder. However, it is not essential to have either HLA DR4 or DRB1*0407 to develop AP.[3]

Clinical presentation

Characteristically patients complain of a perennial problem, with deterioration during the spring and summer months. The relationship to sunlight exposure, however, may not be clear. Pruritus is a prominent feature. The cutaneous response to sunlight has two phases. Following exposure to direct or window-glass transmitted sunlight, pruritic, patchy, edematous erythema with papules and occasionally vesicles develop several hours later. Later, chronic excoriated prurigo lesions are evident often with nodules and plaques. Sometimes eczematization, lichenification, and crusting may occur. The lesions heal leaving postinflammatory scarring and, on the face, small pitted or linear scars may form. The eruption occurs maximally on exposed sites, such as face, ears, dorsal hands, forearms, and lower legs (80–86). Covered sites, for example buttocks, are also frequently affected. The reason for involvement of covered sites remains unclear and cannot be explained by UV penetration through clothing. Unlike PLE, sparing of chronically exposed sites, such as face and back of hands, is unusual. In addition, a history of improvement as the summer progresses is rare. Of diagnostic value, involvement of the distal third of the nose, cheilitis, in particular the lower lip, and conjunctivitis are frequently observed in AP. The latter two features appear to be more commonly reported in Native Americans. Additionally in this group, pterygium formation, thickening of the skin and loss of hair from the eyebrows are common features.

Investigations

The diagnosis of AP is based on the history, clinical features and exclusion of other photodermatoses. Monochromator phototesting is normal in one-third of cases. Abnormal delayed erythemal responses in the UVB and UVA wavelengths are present in approximately two-thirds of cases. Repetitive UVA provocation testing induces lesions in the majority of cases.

Circulating antinuclear factor, anti-SSA (Ro) and anti-SSB (La) titers, plasma porphyrin scan, as well as hematology and biochemistry are normal or negative. HLA tissue typing is useful in cases where the diagnosis is otherwise unclear. The presence of HLA DR4, and in particular its subtype DRB1*0407, while not diagnostic, provides supportive evidence for a diagnosis of AP.

Histology
Histology is often non-specific (see Chapter 15). There is variable hyperkeratosis, acanthosis, spongiosis, and a superficial perivascular lymphohistiocytic cell infiltrate. The features in the chronic stages may show secondary changes of excoriation and features of lichen simplex chronicus in the prurigo-like areas.

Management

Management of AP is generally more difficult when compared with that of PLE. The regular use of a broad-spectrum, high-factor sunscreen and behavioral sunlight avoidance, such as wearing a broad-brimmed hat, appropriate long-sleeved clothing, and avoiding the mid-day sun, remain important as preventive measures. In addition, the application of a UV-protective film on windows at home and on car windows may help. For suppression of acute episodes, potent topical or oral steroids have been used effectively.

Prophylactic narrowband (TL-01) UVB and PUVA desensitization in springtime, given as for PLE, has been shown to be of benefit. Treatment should be restricted to exposed sites and in severely affected individuals, the use of a potent topical steroid to treated sites immediately after UV exposure may help to reduce provocation of AP flares.

Several investigators have reported the successful use of thalidomide in AP but recurrences are common when treatment is discontinued. The high incidence of adverse effects, such as peripheral neuropathy and teratogenicity, particularly in the young female population, does limit its use. A number of other systemic agents have been tried, such as chloroquine, beta-carotene, tetracycline, vitamin E and azathioprine. A lack of consistent benefit in anecdotal observations suggests further work is required to confirm efficacy.

References
1. Lopez Gonzalez G. Solar prurigo. Arch Argent Dermatol 1961;**11**:301–18.
2. Ménagé H du P, Vaughan RW, Baker CS et al. HLA-DR4 may determine expression of actinic prurigo in British patients. *J Invest Dermatol* 1996;**106**:362–4.
3. Dawe RS, Collins P, Ferguson J, O'Sullivan A. Actinic prurigo and HLA-DR4. *J Invest Dermatol* 1997;**108**:233–4.
4. Grabczynska SA, McGregor JM, Kondeatis E, Vaughan RW, Hawk JL. Actinic prurigo and polymorphic light eruption: common pathogenesis and the importance of HLA-DR4/DRB1*0407. *Br J Dermatol* 1999;**140**:232–6.

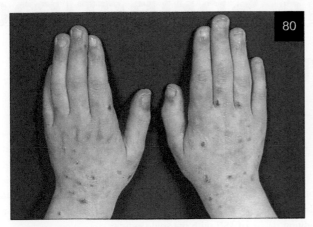

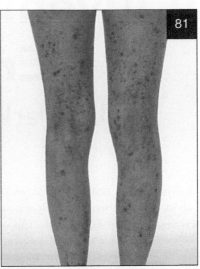

80: Typical excoriated papules on dorsal hands.

81: Prurigo lesions on legs.

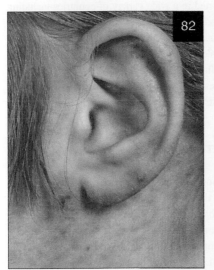

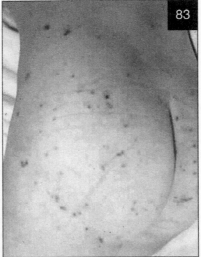

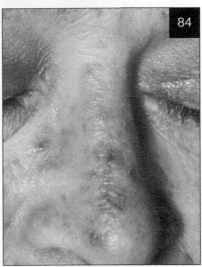

82: Involvement of the ear.

83: Covered site involvement on buttocks.

84: Excoriated and crusted papules on nose.

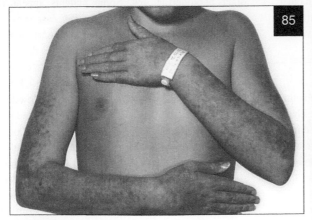

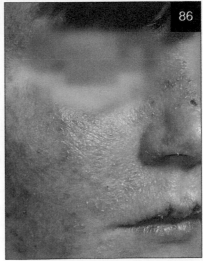

85: Erythematous papules affecting exposed sites on arms with cut-off at the deltoid area.

86: Eczematous AP with involvement on nose and cheilitis.

10 Juvenile Springtime Eruption

Colin Clark and Alyson Bryden

Juvenile springtime eruption (JSE) is a localized idiopathic photodermatosis that typically occurs in spring, affects the ears of young boys, and may occur in outbreaks.[1] This condition, also known as juvenile spring eruption of the ears, juvenile spring eruption or spring eruption of the ears, is seldom reported within the dermatologic literature but is thought to be more common than this would suggest.[2,3]

Epidemiology

Incidence

The true incidence of JSE is unknown, but because of the self-limiting nature of the disorder it may be significantly under-reported and the prevalence could be much higher than previously considered. A survey of New Zealand primary school children on a single occasion in spring found a prevalence of JSE of 12% in young males, and an overall prevalence of 6.7%. The authors concluded that JSE was a relatively common photodermatosis amongst male primary school children in Dunedin, New Zealand.[3]

Age of onset

JSE is classically seen in young boys between the ages of 5 and 12 years.[4] Less commonly it can occur or persist in older teenagers and adults and, unusually, an outbreak in Spain involved a group of male soldiers on military maneuvers in Valencia, aged between 18 and 25 years.

Sex distribution

JSE is more common in boys although the reasons for this male preponderance remain unclear. A class of Swiss school children consisting of 50 boys and 50 girls was studied during fine spring weather and it was found that 44 boys developed typical JSE, whereas only one of the girls was found to have the condition.[5] A short hairstyle and protuberant ears (75th centile or greater) have been strongly associated with the occurrence of JSE, which may be an important factor in the higher prevalence of the disorder in boys. However, a number of young girls with short hair and protuberant ears were also studied and none was found to have the condition.[3] Other etiologic factors may, therefore, be involved in the association of JSE with the male gender.

Geographic distribution

JSE has been reported in a wide variety of countries including the UK, Switzerland, Spain, France, and New Zealand. A recent review of the idiopathic photodermatoses in a Greek photobiology clinic found a prevalence of 4.1% among their patients, indicating that it is not confined to countries with temperate climates. Additionally, studies thus far have failed to demonstrate an association between JSE and either skin tone or hair color.[3]

Mechanism

Although the pathogenesis of JSE is currently unknown, few would question the etiologic role of ultraviolet light. However, monochromatic phototesting is typically normal and the action spectrum for JSE remains elusive. Some authors consider JSE to simply be a localized variant of polymorphic light eruption (PLE),[4] but we believe it has sufficiently characteristic clinical features to merit its distinction from other photodermatoses. Some patients appear to have a genetic predisposition and in one JSE case series a positive family history of the condition was demonstrated in 13 of 18 patients. Another curious feature of JSE is the occurrence of outbreaks, although to date no infectious cause has been identified. The first reported outbreak in the UK was in 1953 when a children's camp in Surrey had to be closed prematurely as a contagious infectious disease was suspected when 121 of 150 children there developed pruritic lesions on their ears. No infectious agent was isolated during this outbreak and it was concluded that environmental factors – the combination of bright sunlight and cold air on exposed sites – were responsible for the eruption. A similar incident was reported in 18 patients in Switzerland in 1942,[5] and a further outbreak occurred amongst a company of Spanish soldiers. Some cases of JSE have resembled erythema multiforme both clinically and histologically, which has led some authors to suggest that JSE may represent a photo-induced variant of erythema multiforme,[5] although others have found no link.[4]

Clinical presentation

Within hours of sunlight exposure, typically in spring, the characteristic eruption appears bilaterally over the helices of the ears. The young boy, usually with short hair and protuberant ears, develops erythematous pruritic papules (1–3 mm) and vesicles over the light-exposed helix (**87**). In more severe cases, JSE will progress from a papular eruption to diffuse erythematous edema, and vesiculation will subsequently evolve to bullae formation and crusting (**88–90**). In the majority of patients, the light-exposed parts of the ears are solely affected; however, the dorsum of the hands may also be involved in some cases.[4] The lesions usually resolve without scarring over 1–2 weeks, if further sunlight exposure is avoided. Although the eruption usually starts in spring, problems can persist throughout the summer months if sunlight exposure is continued.[4]

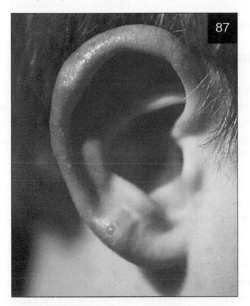

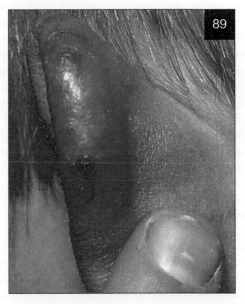

87: Papules and vesicles over the photo-exposed areas of the helix.
88: Diffuse erythema and edema.

89: Erythema, edema and crusting.
90: Erosions and crusting in the healing phase.

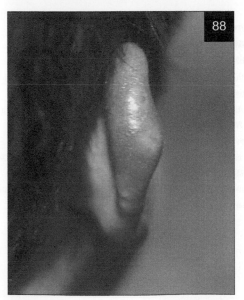

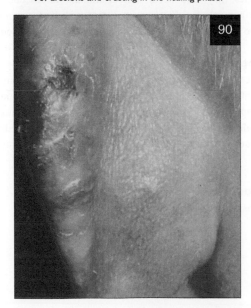

Differential diagnoses

Differential diagnoses of JSE include polymorphic light eruption (PLE), erythema multiforme, hydroa vacciniforme, actinic prurigo, and porphyria. PLE shares a number of features with JSE in that it presents as an itchy, papular eruption several hours after sunlight exposure, has a familial tendency, and has similar non-specific histologic features. It does, however, tend to cause a more generalized eruption and occurs most commonly in young females *(Table 10.1)*. Erythema multiforme is a self-limiting reaction to a broad range of antigenic stimuli and can occur in a photodistributed pattern. Hydroa vacciniforme is an uncommon photodermatosis with a similar age of onset to JSE; however, the eruption is more extensive, usually affecting the cheeks, and resolves with typical varioliform scarring and is rarely restricted solely to the ears. Actinic prurigo should also be considered, but again this condition does not tend to involve the ears in isolation or cause vesicles and blisters, and other characteristic features including distal nose involvement and cheilitis are absent in JSE. Porphyria is unlikely to be confused with JSE and can be readily excluded with a porphyrin plasma scan.

Investigations

Histology

Most patients with this self-limiting condition do not undergo biopsy, but in those that do, the main features are of a predominantly perivascular and periadnexal lymphohistiocytic infiltrate throughout the dermis. Subepidermal spongiotic vesicles may also occur. Direct immunofluorescence has been non-specific. Features consistent with erythema multiforme and polymorphic light eruption have also been observed.[4]

Phototesting

Typically, if performed, monochromatic phototesting in patients with JSE is normal. The use of UVA provocation to attempt to induce the eruption artificially has not been successful, although using solar-simulated radiation repeatedly to produce it may be more useful.[4]

Blood tests

Lupus serology and porphyrin screening are negative.

Table 10.1: **Characteristics of JSE compared with PLE**

Characteristic	JSE	PLE
Sex and age of onset	Young boys	Young adult females
Blistering	Common	Uncommon
Clinical presentation	Uncommon	Common
Prognosis	Usually resolves	Typically persistent
Outbreaks	Yes	No

Management

Most patients with JSE will have a recurring, localized, self-limiting problem occurring annually in the spring, which heals without residual scarring and typically requires no active treatment. Efforts to reduce the frequency and severity of attacks are focused on behavioral sunlight avoidance measures. These include hairstyling, where the hair is allowed to grow longer in order to cover the ears, the use of appropriate clothing such as a broad-brimmed hat, the avoidance of excessive direct sun exposure, i.e. seeking the shade 2 hours either side of the sun's zenith (11am–3pm GMT) and the regular use of an appropriate broad-spectrum high-factor sunscreen. We believe that JSE resolves spontaneously during childhood in the majority of cases, although one case series reported persistence in 6 of 18 patients beyond the age of 12, with one individual still affected at the age of 53.[4]

References

1. Anderson D, Wallace HJ, Howes EIB. Juvenile spring eruption. *Lancet* 1954;i:755–6.

2. Berth-Jones J, Norris PG, Graham-Brown RAC, Burns DA. Juvenile spring eruption of the ears. *Clin Exp Dermatol* 1989;**14**:462–3.

3. Tan E, Eberhart-Phillips J, Sharples K. Juvenile spring eruption: a prevalence study. *NZ Med J* 1996;**109**:293–5.

4. Berth-Jones J, Norris PG, Graham-Brown RAC et al. Juvenile spring eruption of the ears: a probable variant of polymorphic light eruption. *Br J Dermatol* 1991;**124**:375–8.

5. Burckhardt W. Über eine im Frühling, besonders an den Ohren, auftretende Lichtdermatose. *Dermatologica* 1942;**86**:85–91.

11 Photo-aggravated Dermatoses

Robert S Dawe

Many skin diseases can be exacerbated by sunlight exposure. These photo-aggravated dermatoses (PD) differ from the true photodermatoses in that they can also occur without ultraviolet or visible light exposure. The "classic" PDs, such as lupus erythematosus, and other skin diseases that are sometimes photo-aggravated are listed in *Table 11.1*. Only a proportion of those with each of these diseases will report sunlight-induced exacerbations.

Photo-aggravated dermatitis

Epidemiology

Photo-aggravation of dermatitis is best described in atopic dermatitis (**91**). About 10% of people with atopic dermatitis are aware of exacerbations triggered by sunlight. Photo-aggravation has also been noted in seborrheic dermatitis, other endogenous dermatides (especially discoid eczema), and in allergic contact dermatitis.

Mechanism

The mechanisms by which sunlight exposure may exacerbate dermatitis are several. Heat (infrared radiation) effects are probably most important. Irritation by, and in some individuals even IgE-mediated allergy to components of, autologous sweat is one of these factors. Patients may describe sunlight-induced flare-ups, or a dermatitis that is consistently worse in summer than winter, or flaring during phototherapy. Others unaware of a sunlight role present with dermatitis particularly affecting photo-exposed sites suggesting that aggravation by sunlight may be an important environmental factor. A common situation is the patient with a past history of atopic dermatitis, whose dermatitis has recently recurred involving previously unaffected face and photo-exposed chest.

Table 11.1: Photo-aggravated dermatoses

"Classical" photo-aggravated dermatoses	*Other photo-aggravated dermatoses*
• Atopic dermatitis	• Allergic contact dermatitis
• Psoriasis	• Seborrheic dermatitis
• Lupus erythematosus	• Rosacea
• Jessner's lymphocytic infiltrate	• Melasma
• Dermatomyositis	• Mycosis fungoides
• Lymphocytoma cutis	• Vitiligo
• Actinic lichen planus	• Bullous pemphigoid
• Erythema multiforme	• Linear IgA disease
• Acne vulgaris	• Dermatitis herpetiformis
• Pemphigus and chronic benign familial pemphigus	• Chronic ordinary urticaria
• Darier disease and transient acantholytic dermatoses	• Facial telangiectasia
• Disseminated superficial actinic porokeratosis pilaris	• Pityriasis rubra
• Pellagra	• Reticulate erythematous mucinosis
• Viral exanthema, including herpes simplex	• Keratosis pilaris
	• Actinic granuloma

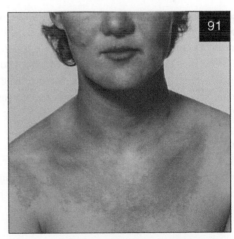

91: The dermatitis distribution here suggested either photo-aggravation or photosensitivity. Negative phototesting excluded true photosensitivity here.

Investigations

It is impossible to diagnose photo-aggravated dermatitis without phototesting to exclude true photosensitivity, particularly the chronic actinic dermatitis syndrome (see Chapter 7). When investigating possible photo-aggravated dermatitis, it is also important to consider the possibility of photo-aggravation from polymorphic light eruption in combination with an endogenous dermatitis. Also, patch testing may be required as contact allergic dermatitis causing exposed site involvement may confuse the situation. If the eyelids are not affected by an exposed site dermatitis, this should raise suspicion of photo-aggravation, true photo-sensitivity or photo-allergy to a sunscreen chemical rather than allergic contact dermatitis. Photo-exposed site discoid eczema has been reported as the presenting feature of porphyria cutanea tarda so a porphyrin plasma scan as screening test for cutaneous porphyria may be appropriate.

Management

Photo-aggravated dermatitis should be managed as for the underlying dermatitis. Phototherapy is often beneficial, although it may be necessary to use lower dose increments than usual.

Photo-aggravated ("photosensitive") psoriasis

The term photo-aggravated psoriasis is used to refer to psoriasis with new lesions occurring, or existing lesions expanding, as a result of sunlight or artificial ultraviolet exposure. This condition is sometimes called "photosensitive psoriasis" although the term "photo-aggravated" is more frequently used for conditions such as this, in which abnormal photosensitivity cannot consistently be demonstrated on objective testing.

Epidemiology

No incidence figures are available for photo-aggravated psoriasis, but the prevalence of photo-aggravation amongst people with psoriasis in Scandinavia is over 5%. It can present at any age, and generally the psoriasis is present before photo-aggravation is noted.

Mechanism

The most common single mechanism for photo-aggravation in psoriasis, at least in countries where polymorphic light eruption (see Chapter 5) is common, is the coincidental development of polymorphic light eruption in someone with pre-existing psoriasis who exhibits the isomorphic (Köbner)

phenomenon (92, 93). Other mechanisms include ordinary sunburn, drug-induced photosensitivity (Chapter 12), lupus erythematosus, and idiopathic photodermatoses other than polymorphic light eruption. Occasionally other photo-aggravated dermatoses, such as Grover's acantholytic dermatosis, also trigger psoriasis through the isomorphic phenomenon. Even after investigation there remain some people in whom the psoriasis photo-induction mechanism remains unclear.

Management

Treatment is as for "ordinary" psoriasis, and the underlying condition. Photo-aggravation of psoriasis is only a contraindication to phototherapy in exquisitely abnormal photosensitivity as a result of one of the more unusual underlying photodermatoses (such as chronic actinic dermatitis or idiopathic solar urticaria), or when lupus erythematosus is diagnosed as the underlying disease. Most patients with photo-aggravated psoriasis can be treated successfully with phototherapy or psoralen photochemotherapy.

Lupus erythematosus

Epidemiology

The prevalence of lupus erythematosus (LE) varies across countries and populations. Systemic LE (SLE) affects around 20/100,000 of the Western European population. Discoid LE and subacute cutaneous LE (SACLE) are more common.

Mechanism

Clinical studies have shown that exacerbation of cutaneous and systemic LE by sunlight is mainly by ultraviolet B and short ultraviolet A (UVA-2, 320–340 nm) wavebands.

Investigations

Cutaneous LE can usually be diagnosed on the basis of the clinical presentation. The morphology of discoid LE lesions, which cause scarring, is characteristic (94). SACLE is occasionally harder to diagnose. Although polymorphic light eruption may be considered on the basis of morphology, LE lesions are usually far more persistent, lasting for months rather than 1–3 weeks. Clinical assessment can be supplemented by skin biopsy and serology (ANA, and anti-Ro and La antibodies).

Clinical presentation

Lupus erythematosus (discoid lupus erythematosus [LE], SCLE, LE tumidus, and SLE with acute cutaneous LE) is often exacerbated by sunlight exposure. Discoid LE (94, 95)

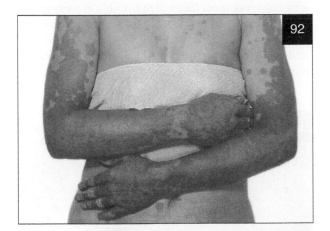

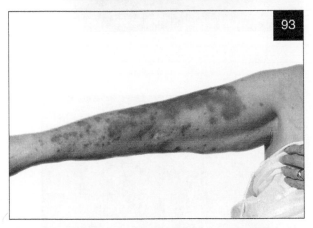

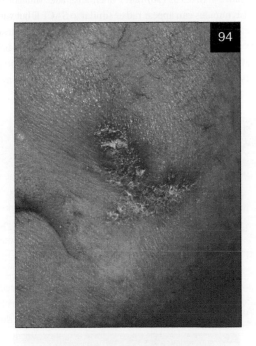

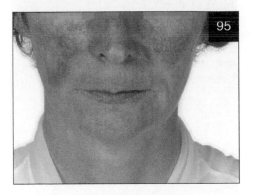

92: Psoriasis confluent on extensor forearms, but with sparing of watch strap-protected area on right wrist. This started as papules of psoriasis following polymorphic light eruption, but lesions have now coalesced.

93: Predominantly photodistributed psoriasis on arm.

94: Note the adherent hyperkeratosis.

95: Largely "burnt-out" CDLE leaving depressed scar on right cheek.

tends to affect chronically sunlight-exposed skin, and some patients note exacerbation of existing lesions after an acute episode of sunlight exposure.

The triggering of new lesions by sunlight is less often reported by DLE patients. SACLE (**96**) flares often arise after sunlight exposure. LE tumidus can appear rather similar to SACLE but without any evidence of any epidermal involvement: SACLE lesions, while initially lacking any features of epidermal involvement, often become scaly. Some cases of Jessner's lymphocytic infiltrate (see below), best considered a reaction pattern that may turn out to have more than one cause, may in fact be tumid LE.

Acute cutaneous LE (**97, 98**), producing the so-called "butterfly rash" across cheeks and bridge of nose, which may also be a feature of other photo-aggravated disorders such as rosacea, can be triggered by sunlight exposure in people presenting with systemic LE (SLE). In SLE, CDLE (**99**) and SACLE may occur as well as the acute cutaneous LE, which is the classic cutaneous feature of SLE. Only a minority (probably 1 in 10 or fewer) of patients who first present with CDLE progress to SLE, but about a third of SACLE patients may subsequently develop SLE. Systemic as well as skin features may flare after sunlight exposure.

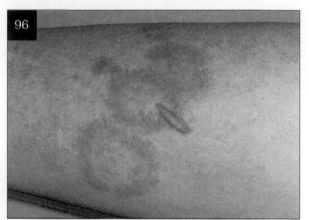

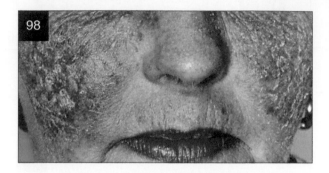

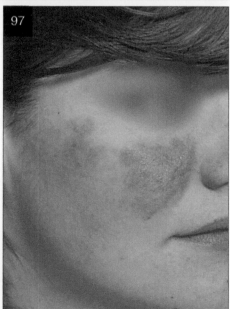

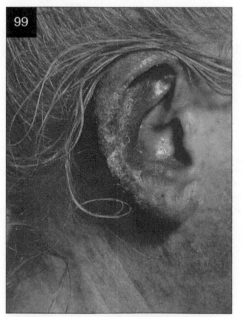

96: This annular pattern is often seen in SACLE (and in Jessner's lymphocytic infiltrate, which can look identical). Note the absence of marked features of epidermal inflammation in this form of cutaneous LE.

97: Dermal inflammation in acute cutaneous LE.

98: Some desquamation evident following an acute sunburn-like flare of acute cutaneous LE in a patient with SLE.

99: Note the adherent hyperkeratosis here in this patient with SLE. Histology may suggest CDLE.

Management

Two small, but well-designed, controlled studies suggested that low-dose ultraviolet A1 (UVA-1, 340–400 nm) phototherapy may be a useful treatment for systemic and cutaneous features of SLE. This is not a standard treatment, but supports the idea that it is the shorter ultraviolet wavebands that cause the patterns of DNA damage involved in exacerbations of LE.

Treatment depends on the pattern of cutaneous lupus, and the presence or absence of systemic (SLE) features. However, all patients should be advised on behavioral and clothing sunlight avoidance measures, supplemented by use of a broad-spectrum, high-factor topical sunblock whether a history of photoprovocation exists or not. Careful advice on photoprotection is especially important for those with DLE, who are not always aware of the role of sunlight. Potent, or very potent, topical steroids are useful, especially in DLE. If these measures are insufficient, hydroxychloroquine may be required. Systemic corticosteroids, and other systemic immunosuppressives, are often necessary for SLE, especially if there is significant systemic involvement.

Jessner's lymphocytic infiltrate

This condition is manifest by erythematous papules or plaques (often shaped as a ring or an arc) (**100, 101**). These is generally asymptomatic. The face, especially cheeks, temples and forehead, are often affected, but a solitary ring on the trunk does not seem uncommon. Lesions are sometimes reminiscent of polymorphic light eruption (see Chapter 5) but tend to persist for weeks or months. These do not leave scars when they eventually resolve. Although aggravation by sunlight is often reported, most patients do not give a clear history of sunlight induction.

Histopathologic features include a dense, or moderately dense, infiltrate of T lymphocytes around both deep and superficial dermal vessels. There may be increased dermal mucin, making the features similar to that of tumid LE. Some consider that Jessner's lymphocytic infiltrate is, in fact, part of the spectrum of cutaneous lupus erythematosus.

Although the only treatment assessed (and found beneficial) in a controlled study was thalidomide, hydroxychloroquine is more commonly prescribed and seems to work (although the evidence base for it is only anecdote).

100: This illustration could equally have been of PLE, but a history of these lesions persisting for many weeks, and exclusion of LE, help to make the diagnosis of Jessner's lymphocytic infiltrate.

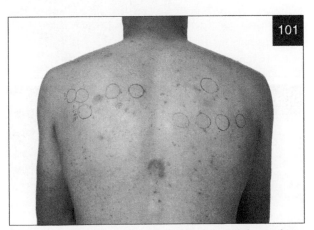

101: Although Jessner's lymphocytic infiltrate is regarded as a photo-aggravated disease and tends to affect photo-exposed sites it is common to see annular or arcuate lesions like this on covered sites of trunk.

Dermatomyositis

Erythema and edema of photo-exposed anterior chest, upper back and back of neck (sometimes called the "shawl sign") is a frequent feature of this disease (**102–104**). Also, a patchy or streaky erythema may be seen on other sunlight-exposed sites. A minority of dermatomyositis patients have demonstrable abnormal photosensitivity on testing. Investigation and treatment of dermatomyositis are essentially the same whether or not photo-aggravation is a feature, although those with definite photo-aggravation should be given advice on behavioral and clothing sunlight avoidance measures. Also, a broad-spectrum, high-factor sunblock may be beneficial.

102: Confluent erythema and edema, with superimposed dermal papules, in dermatomyositis.

103: Note the relative sparing of skin usually covered by bra-straps over shoulders, and the lines of erythema suggesting possible dermographism. This latter feature appears to be common in dermatomyositis, although it is not one of the classic features.

104: The typical dilated nail-fold capillaries and microinfarcts supported the diagnosis in this patient, whose creatine phosphokinase rose to over 5000 from almost normal when she was diagnosed on basis of cutaneous features.

105: Erythemato-telangiectatic rosacea.

Hydroxychloroquine is considered to be more effective for the cutaneous manifestations of dermatomyositis, including those features that are photo-aggravated, than for muscle involvement.

Rosacea

This condition typically affects cheeks, chin, nose and forehead, and is manifest by flushing, telangiectasia and papules and pustules. The most common cases to be exacerbated by sunlight exposure are those where the main features are erythema and telangiectasia (**105**). Sunlight-induced exacerbations mainly involve increased redness, but may lead to increased edema.

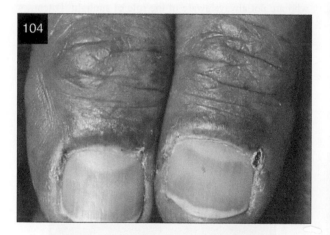

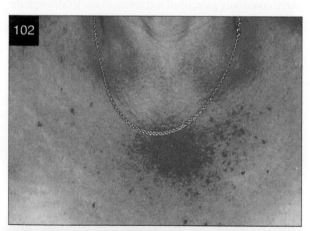

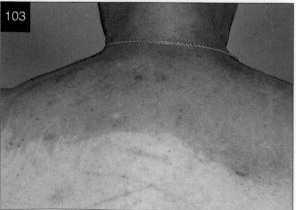

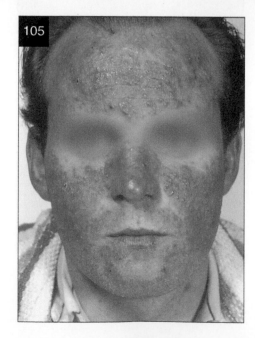

If photo-aggravation appears to be occurring, and new papules appear a few hours after exposure, this might be photo-aggravated rosacea but coincidental polymorphic light eruption should be considered (**106**).

Erythema multiforme

This can sometimes appear upon a sunburn erythema (**107, 108**). It typically affects chronically photo-exposed sites (as well as the "classic" sites of palms, soles, extensor knees, and elbows), even when a clear relationship with sunlight exposure is not noted (**109**). This, the picking out of previously chronically photo-exposed sites, regardless of whether or not photo-aggravation is reported, is also often seen in CDLE.

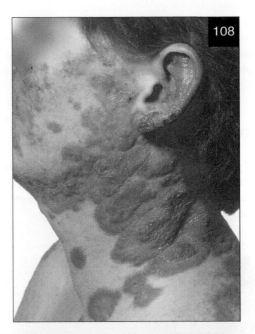

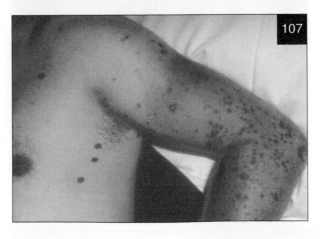

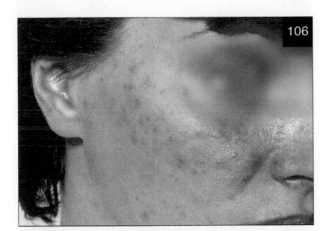

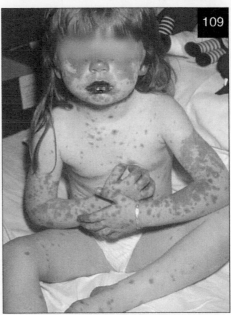

106: Papular polymorphic light eruption in a patient with mild rosacea.
107: Erythema multiforme arising on a mild sunburn.
108: Erythema multiforme on sun-exposed back of neck.
109: Erythema multiforme, secondary to herpes simplex virus infection, in a child. Previously maximally photo-exposed sites are particularly affected; she has not had a recent sunburn.

Mycosis fungoides

Photo-aggravation in this condition (**110**) is uncommon, and phototesting is required to exclude the true photosensitivity of the actinic reticuloid form of chronic actinic dermatitis (see Chapter 7), which can easily be misdiagnosed, on histopathologic and clinical grounds, as mycosis fungoides.

Lymphocytoma cutis

This, probably reactive rather than neoplastic, focal dermal lymphocyte proliferation (**111**) may be photo-aggravated, and has also been noted to accompany polymorphic light eruption and idiopathic solar urticaria.

Actinic lichen planus

This condition (**112, 113**) has been reported mainly in people from the Middle East, East Africa and India. Whether this should be considered a distinct entity or a photodistributed form of ordinary lichen planus remains controversial.

Melasma

This common, usually sharply demarcated, hypermelanosis of forehead, upper lip, cheeks and chin is seen mainly in women, but is not uncommon in men from the Indian subcontinent. It becomes more apparent after sunlight exposure.

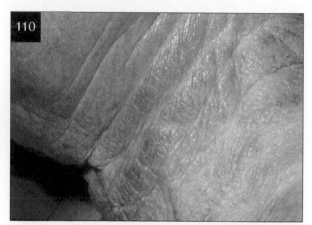

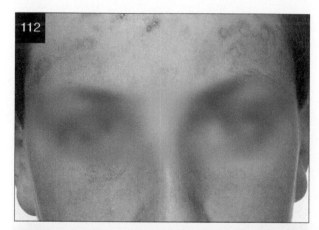

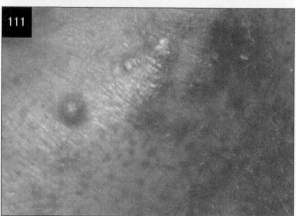

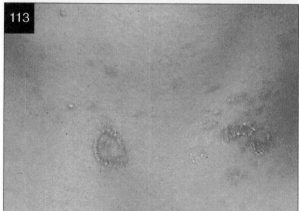

110: Mycosis fungoides on neck with sparing of relatively shaded skin creases. True photo-aggravated mycosis fungoides is rare, and a more common cause for this appearance is the pseudo-reticuloid change that can occur in chronic actinic dermatitis.

111: Lymphocytoma cutis: firm skin-colored and pink papules on maximally photo-exposed site of cheek.

112: Resolving actinic lichen planus, with small rings of hyperpigmentation.

113: More active actinic lichen planus.

Acne vulgaris

Most cases of apparent photo-aggravation of acne vulgaris are probably flares due to heat and humidity. Some reports of "Mallorca acne" may in fact describe solar folliculitis, a rare undefined member of the idiopathic photodermatoses.

Pellagra

Niacin deficiency (usually due to insufficient dietary intake) causes the classic "3Ds" of dermatitis, diarrhea, and dementia, and if untreated progresses to the fourth "D" of death. The "dermatitis" is not a dermatitis and appears as a sunburn-like eruption followed by pigmentation on front of neck and sometimes face.

Others (Table 11.1)

Photo-aggravation of vitiligo is typically due to the Köbner phenomenon, and does not preclude phototherapy or PUVA if otherwise indicated, but warrants great care to avoid causing sunburn-type erythema. Actinic granuloma (see Chapter 15), disseminated superficial porokeratosis, and reticulate erythematous mucinosis tend to pick out chronically photo-exposed sites, but a description of exacerbation by sunlight is usually not forthcoming. Sunlight-induced recrudescence or dissemination of viral infections such as herpes simplex, and of seborrheic dermatitis (in which Mallasezia yeasts are important), is probably due to local immunosuppression. The primary mechanism for photo-aggravation when it occurs in the other disorders in the box not dealt with individually is probably infrared (heat) exacerbation.

Further Reading

1. Frain-Bell, W., Chapter 3. Photoaggravated dermatoses, in Cutaneous photobiology, W. Frain-Bell, Editor. 1985, *Oxford University Press: Oxford*. p. 60-73.

2. Kuhn, A., et al., Lupus erythematosus tumidus--a neglected subset of cutaneous Lupus erythematosus: report of 40 cases. *Arch Dermatol*, 2000. **136**(8): p. 1033-41.

3. Wong, S.N. and L.S. Khoo, Analysis of photodermatoses seen in a predominantly Asian population at a photodermatology clinic in Singapore. *Photodermatol Photoimmunol Photomed*, 2005. **21**(1): p. 40-4.

12 Drug-induced Photosensitivity

James Ferguson

The majority of mild cases of drug-induced photosensitivity either pass unnoticed or are assumed to have been a mild sunburn episode. An increasing number of new drugs that have coincidental photosensitivity are being detected by preregistration drug screening.[1]

Within dermatology clinical practice, the opportunity to apply preventative action should not be missed. Where agents produce photosensitivity by an idiosyncratic mechanism (that is, the great majority of patients taking a particular drug are unaffected), it is more likely that the clinical link with the drug will be missed preregistration, and only be detected by postmarketing surveillance and case reporting.

A number of drug families and individual agents have the ability to change a patient's sensitivity to solar and/or artificial sunlight (*Table 12.1*). While nearly two-thirds of all drugs have the ability to absorb in the ultraviolet region, the great majority of these dissipate the energy in a clinically harmless fashion. Only those that produce a damaging cutaneous effect are described in this chapter.

Mechanism

Drugs induce photosensitivity by a variety of mechanisms (*Table 12.2*).[2] The most common by far of these is phototoxicity, which occurs in many forms and is drug specific in wavelength dependency, timing of onset, and clinical morphology (*Table 12.3*). Other less common mechanisms include lupus erythematosus, lichen planus, pellagra, erythema multiforme, and photo-allergy. Essentially these are of an idiosyncratic type with only a small number of individuals affected for reasons as yet unclear. Although phototoxicity is classically defined as occurring in any individual who is exposed to enough of the drug and appropriate irradiation, there are also idiosyncratic phototoxic agents that, as with the less common mechanisms,

affect only a minority of subjects. A wide variety of drugs have been reported (*Table 12.1*).

Table 12.1: Drugs responsible for photosensitivity

Photosensitizing drugs
- Antibiotics
- Fluoroquinolones
- Nalidixic acid
- Tetracyclines
- Sulfonamides

Antifungals
- Griseofulvin

Diuretics and cardiovascular agents
- Thiazides
- Frusemide
- Amiodarone
- Quinidine

Non-steroidal anti-inflammatory drugs
- Naproxen
- Tiaprofenic acid
- Piroxicam
- Azapropazone

Calcium channel antagonists
- Nifedipine
- Benoxaprofen
(now discontinued)

Psoralens

Psychoactive drugs
- Phenothiazines (chlorpromazine, thioridazine)
- Protriptyline

Retinoids
- Isotretinoin
- Acitretin

Photodynamic therapy agents
- Foscan
- Photofrin

Table 12.2: Mechanisms of drug- and chemical-induced photosensitivity

- Phototoxicity
- Pseudoporphyria
- Photo-allergy
- Lupus erythematosus
- Lichenoid reactions
- Pellagra

Phototoxicity

The most common mechanism by far for the induction of photosensitivity is phototoxicity. The range of clinical presentations *(Table 12.3)* relates to phototoxic drug/metabolite accumulation at different subcellular sites, often multiple. It is known, for example, that some phototoxic drugs target the nucleus, some target cell membranes and mitochondria, and others target lysosomes. It also seems likely that some agents may concentrate at the dermal–epidermal junction, producing fragility in that structure as one of the many patterns of cutaneous phototoxicity with which we are now familiar. With such a range of photochemical events, study is needed to explain the reported variety. In the past, an oversimplification of phototoxicity has clouded the issue. They are not simply exaggerated sunburn events induced by UVA wavelengths. In fact, the major patterns of cutaneous phototoxicity show a range of symptons and signs, as illustrated in *Table 12.3*.

Table 12.3: **Major patterns of cutaneous phototoxicity**

Skin reactions	Photosensitizers
Prickling or burning during exposure; immediate erythema; edema or urticaria with higher doses; sometimes delayed erythema or hyperpigmentation	Photofrin; amiodarone; chlorpromazine
Exaggerated sunburn	Fluoroquinolone antibiotics; chlorpromazine; amiodarone; thiazide diuretics; quinine; demethyl-chlortetracycline and other tetracyclines
Late-onset erythema; blisters with slightly higher doses; hyperpigmentation only with low doses	Psoralens
Increased skin fragility with blisters from trauma (pseudoporphyria)	Nalidixic acid; frusemide; tetracycline; naproxen; amiodarone; fluoro-quinolone antibiotics
Photo-exposed site telangiectasia	Calcium channel antagonists

Clinical presentation

Examination of a patient who may or may not be aware of photosensitivity should focus on the clinical distribution. The photosensitive sites of the face should be examined, looking closely for involvement of the forehead, cheeks, chin, and rim/lobe of ears. The hands may be affected with a "V"-shaped area close to the base of the thumb with sometimes the proximal phalanx involved and sparing between the fingers and distal two-thirds of the dorsum of fingers.

Persistent light reaction

This term describes the continuing state of photosensitive dermatitis. It is believed to follow an initial chemical- or drug-associated photo-allergic episode. It is likely to be rare. Many cases probably represent chronic actinic dermatitis (see Chapter 7).

Investigations

Diagnostic phototesting, best conducted with the monochromator, reveals an abnormality, which will normalize following drug withdrawal. The time to improvement will vary from drug to drug, as will the wavelength of induction. Although the majority of drugs have a UVA dependence, this often extends into the UVB or visible regions. Repeat phototesting off drug should help confirm the diagnosis providing there is improvement towards normal.

Photo-allergy to systemically taken drugs appears rare. Topical non-steroidal anti-inflammatory (NSAID) agents are probably the most important group, although a number of reported reactions may be phototoxic or photo-aggravated in nature. Usage of topical NSAIDs, although increasing throughout Europe as a whole, seems particularly common in Spain, Portugal, and Italy.

Commonly encountered phototoxic drugs

Drug-induced photosensitivity skin reactions can be anticipated with a wide range of agents.

Amiodarone (114)

Amiodarone is a cardiac antidysrhythmic agent with a wide range of phototoxic effects. Acute episodes are commonly high drug dose related with patients presenting with an immediate burning, prickling sensation coupled with erythema which often settles, re-emerging by 24 hours. The problem appears to be common with an incidence of 40–60% primarily in those taking high daily doses. The phenomenon is UVA and visible wavelength dependent and accordingly can occur during the winter months in Europe and can also be induced by window glass-transmitted light, even on cloudy days. The drug has a very long half-life and can persist in the skin for many months. An unusual chronic skin feature, affecting a minority of patients, is a golden-brown pigmentation or an unsightly slate-gray form (115). After stopping the drug, pigmentation and susceptibility to photosensitivity continue for months or even years. For many patients for whom this agent is the drug of last resort, drug cessation is not an option. They usually have to manage with drug dosage reduction and photoprotection.

Phenothiazine (116)

Chlorpromazine, which is still occasionally used as a major tranquillizer, produces a UVA and drug dose-dependent immediate skin discomfort with erythema and blistering. As with amiodarone, golden or unpleasant slate-gray skin pigmentation may occur. Interestingly, drug metabolites may be more phototoxic than the mother compound.

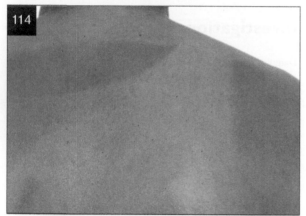

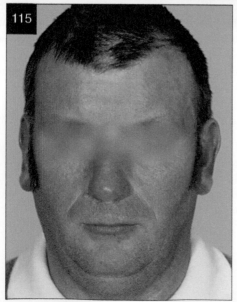

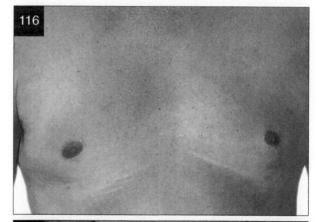

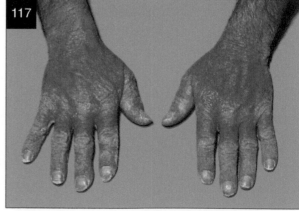

114: Amiodarone phototoxicity as shown by an erythema induced through thin clothing.

115: Slate-gray pigmentation as a complication of amiodarone phototoxicity.

116: Chlorpromazine 200 mg/day followed by sunlight exposure produced this springtime immediate painful erythema, which persisted.

117: Thiazide diuretic-associated phototoxicity affecting the back of hands and proximal phalanges.

Thiazide diuretics (117)

These are agents which are chemically derived from the sulfonamide molecule (also known as a photosensitizer). Phototoxicity is idiosyncratic with the great majority of patients taking the drug having no detectable photosensitivity. In a few, a cutaneous sunburn timescale-type reaction will occur, which, if recurrent, can simulate chronic actinic dermatitis. A lupus and lichen planus-like eruption can arise rarely in some patients. When severe photosensitivity develops, it is best to substitute a relatively non photo-active alternative such as the chemically unrelated loop diuretic, bumetanide. Diagnosis can be established by phototesting which, following drug withdrawal, will gradually normalize over 6 months.

Retinoids

Both roaccutane and etretinate have been reported to induce phototoxic responses in a few individuals (**118**). These can be severe with a broad ultraviolet wavelength dependency. Normalization of the photoresponse occurs within weeks.

Non-steroidal anti-inflammatory agents

One of the most commonly incriminated phototoxic groups, the NSAIDs are capable of provoking reactions in an idiosyncratic fashion. Particular culprits include naproxen, piroxicam (**119**), tiaprofenic acid and ketoprofen. Occasionally, pseudo-porphyria with skin fragility and blistering may arise in addition to phototoxicity, which is characterized by immediate erythema/urticaria followed by delayed erythema. The classic agent in this group studied in the 1980s was benoxaprofen. The majority of patients taking this agent experienced a burning protoporphyria-like discomfort which on phototesting showed an urticaria response accompanied in some by photo-onycholysis and milia (**120**).

Tetracyclines

The classic dimethyl-chlortetracycline phototoxicity is now, owing to infrequent use, rarely encountered. Minocycline appears relatively non-phototoxic. The use of this agent has declined in recent years with many patients now using doxycycline. This drug at high dosage (>200 mg/day) may cause a phototoxic response. The majority of patients taking 100 mg/day seem relatively free of problems.

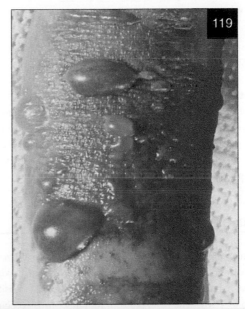

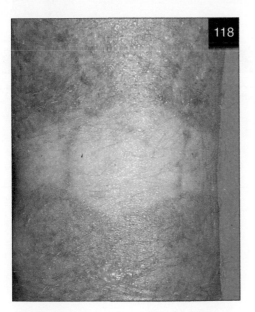

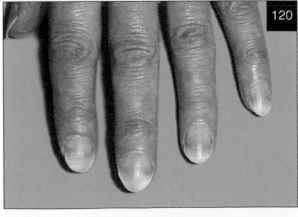

118: Phototoxicity in early springtime following a course of oral Tigason.

119: Piroxicam phototoxicity 48 hours post window glass irradiation. Note the protection by the patient's sandal strap.

120: Photo-onycholysis associated with benoxaprofen phototoxicity.

Quinine

This agent, which is typically taken for the prevention of night leg cramps, can in an idiosyncratic fashion cause a leukomelanoderma (**121**) following a severe erythema. The problem can be induced by UVB and UVA wavelengths. Clearance of the susceptibility may take many months after stopping therapy.

Fluoroquinolone antibiotics

This large group of fluorinated quinolones shows a spectrum of phototoxicity. This tends to have a 24-hour delayed onset with erythema/blistering (**122**) caused by UVA and occasionally visible wavelengths. The phenomenon is molecule specific with minor changes around the quinolone ring associated with a marked alteration in phototoxic potential as measured using the phototoxic index (PI):

$$PI = \frac{\text{baseline predrug MED dose}}{\text{on drug MED dose}}$$

Some members of the family, for example clinafloxacin, have a PI of 100 whereas others appear to photoprotect (**123**).

Photodynamic therapy agents

Photofrin and Foscan are systemic anticancer drugs administered intravenously with subsequent laser irradiation via optical fibers producing tumor cell death. These agents, which can persist in the circulation for several months, can result in severe visible light phototoxic skin reactions (**124**).

Management

Treatment involves substitution by non photo-active alternatives and the use of broad-spectrum sunscreens and sunlight avoidance. Several photo-active drugs can continue to cause photosensitivity for up to 1 year. The main problem for clinicians is recognition of idiosyncratic drug events, which requires constant awareness.

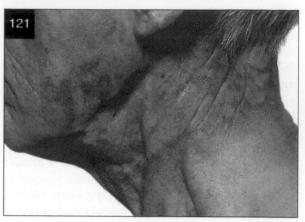

121: Melanomaleukoderma as a consequence of quinine phototoxicity.

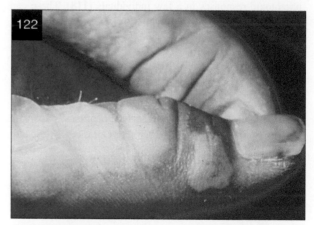

122: An experimental fluoroquinolone was responsible for this severe blistering phototoxicity of back of hands/fingers.

References

1. Ferguson J. Drug and chemical photosensitivity. In: Hawk JLM, ed. *Photodermatology.* London: Arnold Publishers, 1999.

2. Harber LC, Bickers DR. Drug-induced photosensitivity (phototoxic and photo-allergic drug reactions). *In: Photosensitivity Diseases: Principles of Diagnosis and Treatment,* 2nd ed. Toronto: B.C. Decker, 1989.

3. Barratt MD. Structure-activity relationships and prediction of the phtotoxic and phototoxic potential of new drugs. *Alternatives to Laboratory Animals* 2004; **32**: 511-524.

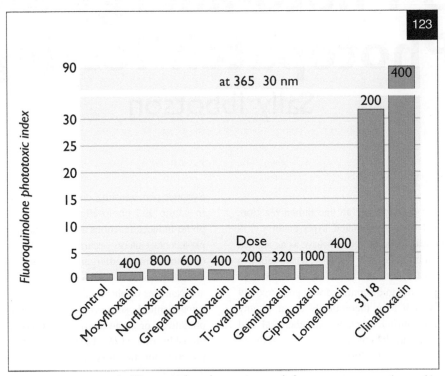

123: Phototoxic potential of fluoroquinolone drugs varies greatly from one agent to another as this phototest-derived phototoxic index demonstrates.

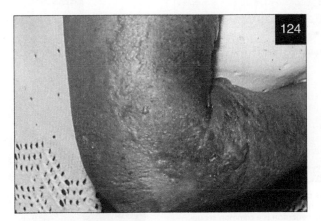

124: Photofrin injection for the management of lung cancer can be responsible for severe phototoxic skin reactions, weeks or even months after injection.

13 Photo-allergy and Photopatch Testing

Sally Ibbotson

Photo-allergy

Photo-allergic contact dermatitis is an uncommon reaction, thought to be caused by cell-mediated hypersensitivity. A photo-activated chemical is considered to behave as an antigen or hapten, eliciting an immunologic response, which requires ultraviolet irradiation for both the induction and elicitation phases. Photo-allergy is not to be confused with phototoxicity (see Chapter 12), which may theoretically occur in any individual exposed to sufficient phototoxic chemical and light of the appropriate wavelength, and which is considered to be a non-immunologic event (125).

Systemic photosensitive drug eruptions are typically phototoxic in nature and photo-allergy is rarely implicated. Topical photo-induced reactions are most commonly phototoxic, with photocontact allergy occurring much less frequently. Examples of photocontact allergens are musk ambrette and para-aminobenzoic acid (PABA), whereas psoralens and porphyrins are examples of phototoxic agents (*Table 13.1*). Interestingly, some chemicals, such as chlorpromazine, are capable of eliciting phototoxic or photo-allergic reactions, although the latter is probably rare (126, 127). Photopatch testing should be reserved for the investigation of suspected photocontact

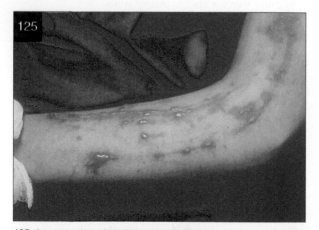

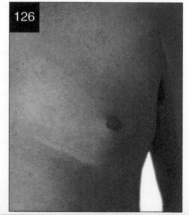

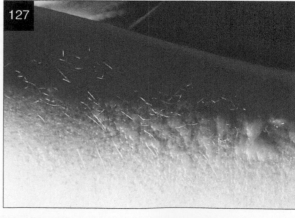

125: An acute phytophotodermatitis caused by psoralen phototoxicity after giant hogweed contact and sunlight exposure. Note the linear pattern and acute blistering. Hyperpigmentation is a common sequel.
126, 127: Photosensitivity in a patient taking systemic chlorpromazine (126). Note the acute blistering (127).

Table 13.1: **Examples of phototoxic agents**

- Psoralens
- Porphyrins
- Phenothiazines, for example chlorpromazine
- Non-steroidal anti-inflammatory drugs,
  for example ketoprofen
- Tar/pitches
- Dyes, for example benzanthrone, acridine orange

allergy and should not be routinely used for the investigation of phototoxic reactions or systemic drug photosensitivity.

Mechanisms

The mechanism of photocontact allergy is not fully understood. Photo-allergy is most widely considered to reflect a delayed-type IV cell-mediated immune response and may have several clinical manifestations, although typically presents as a dermatitis. It does not occur on first exposure to the photo-allergen and its clinical features may include spread beyond the original exposure site. Elicitation is by very low doses of irradiation of the appropriate wavelength, in keeping with an immune reaction. In contrast, drug phototoxicity may occur on first exposure and usually presents as an exaggerated sunburn reaction, rather than a dermatitis process. Photocontact allergy also differs histologically from phototoxicity, with vesicle formation, epidermal spongiosis, and a dermal perivascular mononuclear cell infiltrate typically occurring in the former, whereas epidermal toxicity, edema, and necrosis are features of the latter.

Thus, the clinical and histologic features of photocontact allergy simulate those of allergic contact dermatitis. Photocontact sensitization to photo-allergens, such as chlor-promazine and the halogenated salicylanilides, has been shown in humans and in animal models. Furthermore, passive transfer studies also support the hypothesis of a delayed hypersensitivity reaction as the basis for photocontact allergy.

So the most plausible hypothesis for photocontact allergy is that of absorption of ultraviolet radiation by the chemical, such that the photoproduct acts as antigen or hapten and attaches to a carrier protein, initiating an immune response. Indeed, the modification of histidines in human serum albumin was demonstrated when tetrachlorosalicylanilide (TCSA) was irradiated in the presence of this protein. It appears that this phenomenon is specific and not all proteins in the skin are capable of acting as carriers for antigen or hapten in photocontact allergy.

A state of continuing photosensitivity after an acute episode of photocontact allergic dermatitis to several photocontact allergens, including musk ambrette and buclosamide, has been described, despite the absence of continued chemical exposure. Patients developed acute photocontact allergy, with positive photopatch tests and initially with sensitivity in the UVA region but subsequently development of UVB photosensitivity, with persistence for months or years despite no further allergen exposure. These patients were labeled as persistent light reactors. It was proposed that the persistent light reactor state reflected retention of minute amounts of the photocontact allergen in skin. However, induction of persistent light reactivity in a guineapig model after photo-allergen exposure supported the hypothesis of this reflecting modification of endogenous carrier protein by ultraviolet exposure in the presence of antigen or hapten, such that this altered protein was then able to elicit the delayed hypersensitivity reaction in the presence of light, but without further chemical exposure. However, in practice, most of the reported cases of persistent light reactivity were elderly males who would now fit into the diagnostic criteria for chronic actinic dermatitis, and the existence of a state of persistent light reactivity is controversial.

History and background

Photocontact allergic dermatitis was first described following an outbreak in factory workers after handling a soap containing the antibacterial agent TCSA. Indeed, between 1960 and 1962, TCSA produced an estimated 10,000 cases of photosensitivity in England. Subsequently there were many other reports of photocontact allergy to other halogenated salicylanilides and to chlorinated phenol compounds such as bithionol or fentichlor, or the less closely related mixture of buclosamide and salicylic acid (Jadit, Germany). These were antibacterial, antiseptic, and antifungal agents which were added to soaps and other products in the 1960s and 1970s, and were found to be potent causes of both contact and photocontact allergy. Other antibacterial and preservative compounds, such as the carbanilides and hexachlorophene, have additionally been reported to cause photocontact allergy, although less commonly. The use of these compounds therefore diminished, and in the UK these are no longer relevant allergens, being of historic interest only. Musk ambrette subsequently became one of the commonest photocontact allergens in the late 1970s and, in addition, the synthetic fragrance 6-methyl coumarin was also found to be such a potent photocontact allergen that its use in perfume was discontinued. The concentration of musk ambrette used in perfume products was reduced, and since 1994 it has no longer been available in topical preparations manufactured in Europe, although may still be imported from products manufactured elsewhere, such as in Asia.

There are also several diverse compounds that have been reported to cause photocontact allergy, including chlorpromazine, promethazine, diphenhydramine, and olaquindox, a growth promoter added to animal feed and used by pig farmers. However, there is little or no evidence to support some of these reactions as being photo-allergic in nature. For example, there is no evidence that hydrocortisone is a photocontact allergen and, although balsam of Peru and the Compositae may be phototoxic, they are not considered to be photo-allergic in nature *(Table 13.2)*.

At present, the main group of photocontact allergens is the absorbent sunscreen chemicals and these have their own history. The earliest reported episodes of photocontact allergy to sunscreens were to PABA and, to a lesser extent, to the PABA esters. Indeed, contact and photocontact allergy to PABA and its esters were so common that the use of these chemicals was dramatically reduced and they were largely replaced by the benzophenones. This latter group of chemicals then became the commonest group of sunscreen photocontact allergens and oxybenzone (benzophenone 3), in particular, was implicated in many cases, mainly because of its widespread use not only in sunscreen preparations, but also in facial moisturizers. With the development of more efficient UVA-absorbing sunscreen chemicals, such as the dibenzoylmethanes, photocontact allergy to this chemical group has increasingly been reported and it seems likely that, with the ever-changing pattern of exposure to sunscreen chemicals, this will be a rapidly evolving field.

Photopatch testing

Indications
Photopatch testing should be reserved for the investigation and diagnosis of clinically suspected photocontact allergy. Photocontact allergy may occur in patients with normal ultraviolet radiation sensitivity, such as in regular sunscreen users, or may be a secondary problem that develops in patients with existing photosensitivity such as polymorphic light eruption or chronic actinic dermatitis. There has been considerable variation in the methodology for photopatch testing both in the UK and elsewhere in Europe and in the United States. On this basis, the British Photodermatology Group reviewed the subject of photocontact allergy and photopatch testing and published guidelines based on the existing literature and the consensus practice in the UK at that time, in an attempt to standardize the photopatch test technique in the UK. Photopatch testing should be considered in any patient reporting a history of precipitation or aggravation of an eruption by sunlight in association with sunscreen use (**128**) or in patients with either a history of, or current, photo-exposed site dermatitis (**129**). Additionally, in patients with known photosensitivity

Table 13.2: **Chemicals that have been used in photopatch testing**

Antibacterial, antiseptic and antifungal agents (historic interest in the UK)	Fragrance ingredients	Absorbent sunscreen chemicals	Medicaments and drugs	Miscellaneous
Tetrachlorosalicylanilide and other halogenated salicylanilides	Musk ambrette	PABA and esters	Chlorpromazine	Chlorhexidine
Hexachlorophene	6-methyl coumarin	Dibenzoylmethanes, for example Parsol 1789, Eusolex 8020 (withdrawn)	Promethazine	Thiourea
Fentichlor	Sandalwood oil	Benzophenones, for example oxybenzone, mexenone	Diphenhydramine	Olaquindox
Buclosamide	Balsam of Peru	Cinnamates, for example Parsol MCX, Givtan F (withdrawn)	Non-steroidal anti-inflammatory drugs, for example ketoprofen	Diallyl disulfide
Bithionol		Camphor derivatives	Benzocaine	Compositae
Triclosan			Hydrocortisone	Hexamidine

disease, particularly chronic actinic dermatitis, the possibility of photocontact allergy to sunscreen use should be considered if there is an unexplained deterioration of photosensitivity or a change in its nature (**130**). Extra vigilance is required for photosensitive subjects as they are likely to use sunscreens more regularly and the risk of sensitization to photocontact allergens may therefore be increased. However, photopatch testing may be particularly difficult to perform and interpret in this patient group.

Methods
In the UK, photopatch testing is performed either in photobiology units or in centers with contact dermatitis expertise, and the protocols vary accordingly, largely to accommodate whether the patients are phototested or not. A minimal amount of materials and equipment is required and the technique is straightforward. However, the most important aspect of the method is interpretation of the results and, for this, considerable expertise is required.

Equipment
The action spectrum for induction of photocontact allergy is known for very few photo-allergens, although in those studies which have been performed, UVA appears to be the most relevant waveband. There are practical reasons for the use of UVA in that the induction of UVB erythema at doses below those required to elicit photocontact allergy with a UVB source would preclude its use and, in general, UVA is used for routine photopatch testing. Indeed, a recent study indicated that there was no advantage to the additional use of UVB in photopatch testing.

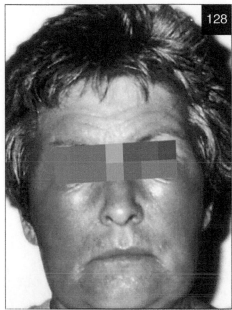

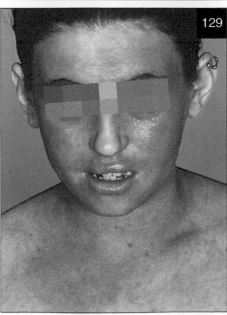

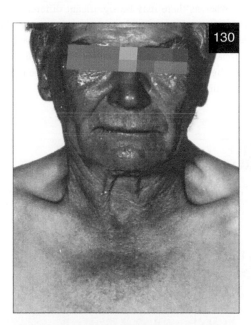

128: Photopatch testing should be performed in a patient with a history of an adverse reaction to sunscreens. Acute facial swelling and erythema occurred in this patient in association with sunscreen use.

129: Photopatch testing was performed in this patient with atopic dermatitis. She had noticed a change in pattern of her dermatitis, with the development of photo-exposed site involvement. She had a history of sunscreen use.

130: This patient with chronic actinic dermatitis was photopatch tested because his photo-exposed site dermatitis deteriorated. He had been using sunscreens.

The characteristics of the UVA source are that it should be a continuous, broadband, well-characterized, and stable output with a uniform and variable field. High irradiance of the source is desirable as this reduces the irradiation times during the procedure. Several UVA sources have been used in photopatch testing, including fluorescent, metal halide, and xenon arc sources, the latter coupled to a monochromator. However, in practice, the fluorescent UVA sources as used in conventional PUVA therapy are typically used, and irradiations can be performed using a free-standing unit (**131**), a mounted hand and foot device, or a whole-body cabinet with the patient appropriately gowned (**132**). The advantage of the use of a xenon arc source coupled to a monochromator is that this allows for flexibility in using low UVA doses when photopatch testing a photosensitive patient, and this may be considered in certain instances in specialized photobiology units, although it is more time consuming as each allergen site must be irradiated separately (**133**).

In general, there is greater consistency between the emission spectra for the fluorescent UVA lamps used in photopatch testing, whereas there may be significant differences in the spectral outputs of metal halide sources. It is essential that the full details of the UVA source used are defined, as discrepancies in photopatch testing results have been shown with the use of different light sources, and the irradiance must be monitored using a calibrated hand-held UVA meter.

There has been a range of UVA doses used for irradiation during photopatch testing, in general 1– 15 J/cm^2, although most of the published literature has reported on the use of either 5 or 10 J/cm^2. Many of the European centers outside the UK have used 10 J/cm^2 and, on reviewing the literature, it is apparent that a high incidence of positive photopatch test results of uncertain relevance is obtained with this dose and is likely to reflect phototoxicity reactions, which are clinically unimportant and are not seen as commonly in those studies

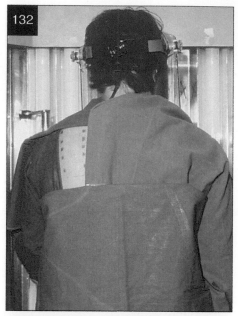

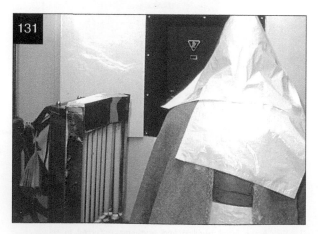

131: Fluorescent UVA lamps, as used in PUVA, can be used for photopatch testing, as shown with this free-standing unit. Note the patient is fully covered, except for the allergen sites to be irradiated.

132: A whole-body UVA cabinet can be used for photopatch testing, as long as the patient is appropriately gowned.

133: A xenon arc lamp coupled to a monochromator can be used for UVA irradiation of photopatch tests in photobiology units. This allows flexibility in delivering low doses of UVA if the patient is photosensitive.

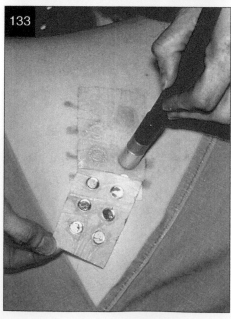

using 5 J/cm². Evidence suggests that it may be possible to reduce the UVA dose to 1 J/cm² or less without the risk of false-negative results. However, in the absence of literature to suggest the contrary, the British Photodermatology Group recommend the use of 5 J/cm² UVA in the standard photopatch test technique in subjects of presumed normal photosensitivity. It is essential that, if photosensitivity is a possibility clinically, a UVA dose series is performed prior to irradiation of the photopatch tests, in order to determine the 24-hour minimal erythema dose. Although there are no firm guidelines, a suberythemogenic dose should be used for irradiation in the photopatch test procedure and a dose of 50% of the UVA MED is commonly used.

Protocols and technique

Allergen series are prepared in the usual way on aluminum Finn chambers in duplicate series (**134**). These are applied to the back (**135**), avoiding the paravertebral area, and after 24 or 48 hours, one set of allergens is removed and assessed and irradiation performed. Patch test readings are performed by standard methods at 48 hours after irradiation and many centers perform additional readings immediately before and after irradiation and at 24 and/or 72 or 96 hours. It is unclear as to whether the period of allergen application prior to irradiation at 24 or 48 hours influences the outcome of photopatch testing, and there is no evidence that either method is superior. In general, centers performing phototesting will often leave allergens in place for 24 hours so that phototesting readings can be performed prior to irradiation, whereas centers with contact dermatitis expertise may use a period of allergen application of 48 hours before irradiation.

The standard dose of 5 J/cm² will be used in the majority of photopatch test procedures, although, if the patient is photosensitive, as mentioned, a suberythemal UVA dose will be used. In some photosensitive patients with extreme UVA photosensitivity, in particular chronic actinic dermatitis, it is not possible to perform or interpret photopatch testing accurately. A high proportion of these patients develop positive photopatch test reactions but the relevance is often not clear. Although there are no clear guidelines, it is also important that, if photopatch testing is performed in a photosensitive patient, topical steroid use at the test sites should be avoided for at least a week before testing if possible, in order to minimize the risk of false-negative results. The effect of systemic immunosuppressants, such as prednisolone, azathioprine or cyclosporin, on photopatch test results is unknown. However, the possibility of false-negative results must be considered, and immunosuppression should be discontinued for at least 1 month before testing if possible.

Interpretation of photopatch testing

It is important to have expertise available for the interpretation of photopatch testing, as this may be difficult, particularly in photosensitive patients. In a straightforward case, interpretation

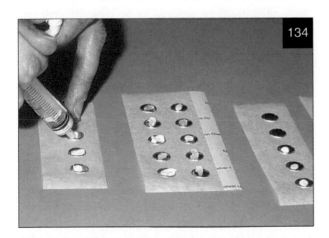

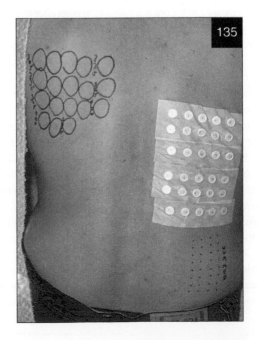

134: Allergen preparation for photopatch testing.
135: Allergen application to the back in duplicate series, avoiding the paravertebral region. Note the patient has also had irradiation monochromator phototesting and a UVA dose series performed.

of results may be obvious. If there is a strong positive reaction on the irradiation site, with a negative control site, this is usually indicative of photocontact allergy (**136, 137**), although the possibility of a phototoxic reaction must also be considered. A strong positive control site indicates the presence of contact allergy (**138**). Weaker reactions can be more difficult to interpret and a diagnosis of phototoxicity or a combination of a suberythemal concentration of irritant or allergen combined with a suberythemal dose of UVA may need to be considered. Indeed, it is possible to induce a false-positive photopatch test result with the combined use of a suberythemal irritant and suberythemal irradiation dose (**139**).

It is of interest that, in the the literature, some centers allow a combined diagnosis of contact allergy with photocontact allergy if the irradiated site response is significantly more positive than that of the control site. However, in general, we would recommend that weak augmentation of a contact site response by irradiation is non-specific and not indicative of photocontact allergy. Furthermore, although uncommon, photosuppression of contact allergy by irradiation can occur, although the significance of this is unclear.

The pattern of response may be important in establishing the nature of the reaction. A crescendo response increasing from the 24-hour reading is usually indicative of a photo-allergic reaction, whereas a decrescendo pattern with reduction in the positive response from 24 hours usually signifies phototoxicity. However, this can only be performed in centers where multiple readings of photopatch tests are performed and is not possible if readings are carried out at a single time point after irradiation.

It may not be possible to interpret the photopatch test technique if the patient develops generalized erythema with irradiation or a reaction to the adhesive tape (**140**). Additionally, if the patient is so exquisitely UVA sensitive that meaningful irradiation may not be possible, contact reactions may be the only ones that can be assessed. Finally, if the result is entirely negative then, although this is likely to indicate that there have been no significant reactions, you need to consider the possibility of technical failure in the methodology. Thus, in interpretation of any photopatch test result it is essential to determine whether the results are of clinical relevance, and a simple assessment of the current relevance of a photo-allergen and the possible route of sensitization is of practical importance.

Which agents should be tested?

Historically, vast numbers of agents have been included in photopatch testing, particularly in the Scandinavian,

Austrian, German, Swiss and American photopatch test series (*Table 13.1*). However, many of these agents, such as halogenated salicylanilides, fragrances, and medicaments and miscellaneous products, such as chlorpromazine, olaquindox, and the non-steroidal anti-inflammatory drugs are either of historic interest only or are considered clinically irrelevant, in view of their phototoxic potential, by those practicing photopatch testing in the UK. Photopatch testing to non-steroidal anti-inflammatories is extensively practiced elsewhere in Europe, but not as commonly in the UK. At present, the absorbent sunscreen chemicals are the major photo-allergen group in the UK and should be included in photopatch testing.

The situation is rapidly evolving and, although the British Photodermatology Group recommended a standard photopatch test series in 1997 (*Table 13.3*), this already appears to have been superseded and is in need of updating, as it is likely that musk ambrette can be discontinued from the photopatch test battery and that several newer sunscreen chemicals need to be considered. Photocontact allergy has been reported to each of the main absorbent sunscreen chemical groups, and it seems that photocontact allergy will represent the sunscreen exposure pattern at any particular time, and as such will require a continuous update.

Several large studies have been performed in order to ascertain the incidence of photocontact allergy in selected patient groups. The results of some of these studies have been complicated by the fact that irradiation doses that may have elicited phototoxic reactions were used and, as such, many of the positive reactions appeared to be clinically irrelevant. Despite the variation in methodology and interpretation, positive photopatch test reactions of the order of approximately 5–10% are commonly reported in these studies.

Problems and variables

It is clear that there are many outstanding issues with photopatch testing, that the methodology is still not standardized, and that many areas need to be clarified. It is likely that a common allergen battery could be considered for use. However, changes in environmental exposure and in the indications for photopatch testing may indicate that supplementary allergen batteries may be required, particularly for use in countries outside the UK. Some of the parameters that require further study are the concentration, vehicle, and duration of allergen application, the wavelength dependency for induction of photocontact allergy for a range of allergens, the UVA source and dose used, timing of irradiation, and interpretation of the data.

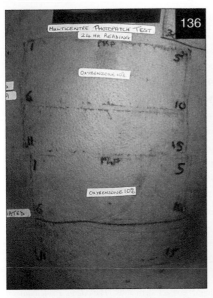

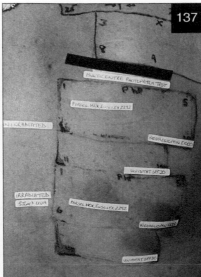

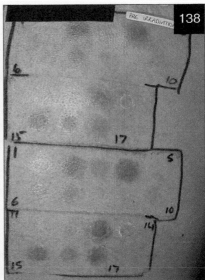

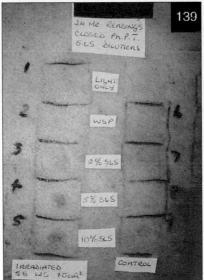

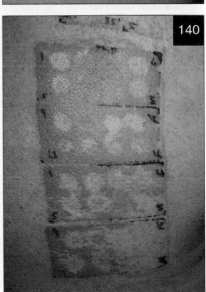

136: A positive photopatch test reaction to oxybenzone (benzophenone 3), a commonly used sunscreen chemical, with a negative unirradiated control site.

137: Multiple positive photopatch tests to sunscreen chemicals, with negative non-irradiated control sites, indicative of photocontact allergy.

138: Multiple positive patch tests to several sunscreen chemicals on both allergen test sites pre-irradiation, indicative of contact allergy.

139: Induction of a false positive photopatch test in the presence of combined suberythemal concentrations of the non-phototoxic irritant, sodium lauryl sulphate and suberythemal doses of ultraviolet irradiation using a solar simulator source.

140: Reaction to adhesive tape obscuring photopatch test sites and resulting in an uninterpretable outcome.

Table 13.3: **Suggested standard series of photo-allergens in 1997 (British Photodermatology Group Guidelines)**

- Para-aminobenzoic acid (PABA)
- Octyl-dimethyl PABA (Escalol 507)
- 2 ethylhexyl-p-methoxycinnamate (Parsol MCX)
- Oxybenzone (benzophenone 3)
- 4-tert-butyl-4-methoxy dibenzoylmethane (Parsol 1789)
- Musk ambrette
- Patient's own product

The use of sunscreens has increased both in subjects of normal sensitivity wishing to prevent sunburn and the long-term risks of excessive ultraviolet radiation exposure and in photosensitive patients whose sunscreen requirements are more specific. Despite these increases in sunscreen use, the incidence of photocontact allergy appears to be low and irritancy and cosmetic unacceptability are more common problems. Indeed, it is more likely that allergy to a sunscreen product is due to the preservatives rather than the sunscreen chemical itself.

The British Photodermatology and Contact Dermatitis Groups have attempted to standardize the indications for photopatch testing, methodology, and interpretation, in order to clarify these issues in selected patient groups. This formed the basis of a prospective multicenter study, which was performed over a 2-year period and has recently been completed and submitted for publication. An expanded allergen battery of 11 candidate sunscreens and the possibility of testing to the patient's own products is included in the study (*Table 13.4*). In the light of these data, information relating to the incidence of photocontact allergy and its clinical relevance in selected patient groups will be available, although this will require a frequent update, in keeping with the changing patterns of photo-allergen exposure both in the UK and elsewhere in Europe. The establishment of a European Taskforce will aim to address these issues.

Table 13.4: **Sunscreen series used in the UK multicenter photopatch test study**

- Para-aminobenzoic acid (PABA)
- Octyl-dimethyl PABA (Escalol 507)
- 2 ethylhexyl-p-methoxycinnamate (Parsol MCX)
- Oxybenzone (Benzophenone 3)
- 4-tert-butyl-4-methoxy dibenzoylmethane (Parsol 1789)
- 3-(4-methylbenzylidene)-camphor (Mexoryl SD)
- 2 hydroxy-4-methoxybenzophenone (Benzophenone 4)
- Isoamyl-p-methoxycinnamate (Neoheliopan)
- 2-phenyl-5-benzimidazolsulfonic acid (Eusolex 232)
- Octyl triazone
- SPF 60 commercial sunscreen product
- Patient's own product

Further reading

Bakkum RSLA, Heule F. Results of photopatch testing in Rotterdam during a 10-year period. *Br J Dermatol* 2002;**146**:275–9.

Bell HK, Rhodes LE. Photopatch testing in photosensitive patients. *Br J Dermatol* 2000;**142**:589–90.

Berne B, Ros AM. 7 Years experience of photopatch testing with sunscreen allergens in Sweden. *Contact Dermatitis* 1998;**38**:61–4.

Bruynzeel DP, Ferguson J, Andersen K, Gonçalo M, English J, Holzle E, Ibbotson SH, Lecha M, Lehmann P, Leonard F, Moseley H, Pigatto P, Tanew A. Photopatch testing: a consensus methodology for Europe. *J Euro Acad Dermatol Venereol* 2004; **18**: 679-682

Darvay A, White IR, Rycroft RJG, Jones AB, Hawk JLM, McFadden JP. Photo-allergic contact dermatitis is uncommon. *Br J Dermatol* 2001;**145**:597–601.

DeLeo VA, Suarez SM, Maso MJ. Photo-allergic contact dermatitis. Results of photopatch testing in New York, 1985 to 1990. *Arch Dermatol* 1992;**128**:1513–18.

English JS, White IR, Cronin E. Sensitivity to sunscreens. *Contact Dermatitis* 1987;**17**:159–62.

Goosens A. Photoallergic contact dermatitis. *Photoderm Photoimmunol Photomed* 2004; **20**: 121-125

Hölzle E, Neumann N, Hausen B et al. Photopatch testing: the 5-year experience of the German, Austrian and Swiss Photopatch Test Group. *J Am Acad Dermatol* 1991;**25**:59–68.

Ibbotson SH, Farr PM, Beck MH et al. British Photodermatology Group. Workshop report: photopatch testing–methods and indications. *Br J Dermatol* 1997;**136**:371–6.

Neumann NJ, Hölzle E, Plewig G et al. Photopatch testing: the 12-year experience of the German, Austrian and Swiss Photopatch Test Group. *J Am Acad Dermatol* 2000;**42**:183–92.

Schauder S, Ippen H. Contact and photocontact sensitivity to sunscreens. *Contact Dermatitis* 1997;**37**:221–32.

Thune P, Jansen C, Wennersten G, Rystedt I, Brodthagen H, McFadden N. The Scandinavian multicenter photopatch study 1980–1985: final report. *Photodermatology* 1988;**5**:261–9.

Wilkinson DS. Photodermatitis due to tetrachlorosalicylanilide. *Br J Dermatol* 1961;**73**:213–19.

14 Phytophotodermatitis
James Ferguson

Although strictly speaking not a dermatitis and in fact more akin to a sunburn reaction, phytophotodermatitis (a term coined in 1942 by Robert Klaber[1]) describes a group of plant- and light-induced combined skin effects. As would be expected, it has a much longer history than modern drug-induced photosensitive reactions.

This group of conditions does not include the persistent light reactor state where plant contact allergy, typically to the Compositae family, can become associated with photosensitivity of a chronic actinic dermatitis (CAD) type. Whether the true concept of persistent light reactor, i.e. that photo-allergy is followed by a persistent photosensitivity state, really exists has not been convincingly proven.

Plants and mechanisms

The naturally occurring chemicals sourced from plants that come in contact with the skin and are subsequently irradiated by sunlight producing the characteristic clinical features are many and varied (Table 14.1).

The same family of chemicals are the furocoumarins, which contain photo-active linear psoralens (8-methoxypsoralen: 8-MOP and 5-MOP) and angelicins. These chemicals have been isolated from a range of plant species including Umbelliferae, Moraceae, Rutaceae, and Leguminosae. Typically, when the sap of such plants is in contact with the skin and subsequently exposed to enough light in the UVA (320–400 nm) region, this will, some 24–72 hours later, induce a raised erythema, blistering, and a chronic brown pigmentation due to melanin deposition.

Historic aspects

Over the last 3000 years, most notably in the Nile, Mesopotamian, and Indus Valley cultures, local knowledge established that an extract of various parts of local plants (for example, *Ammi majus*) was capable, when applied to the skin and subsequently exposed to sunlight on a repeated basis, of treating the depigmentary disorder vitiligo. Scientific study by the remarkable Andalusian botanist and pharmacist Ibn Al Bitar, as early as the 13th century, assessed such parameters as the duration of plant extract application and the dose of sunlight exposure required for the desired therapeutic effect.

Table 14.1: **Plants commonly reported to cause phytophotodermatitis and containing psoralens.**

Order	Botanical name	Common name
Leguminosae	*Psoralea corylifolia*	Bavachee
Umbelliferae	*Ammi majus*	Aatrillal
	Angelica archangelica	Angelica
	Anethum graveolens	Dill
	Apium graveolens	Celery
	Daucus carota	Wild carrot
	Daucus sativa	Garden carrot
	Foeniculum vulgare	Fennel
	Heracleum gigantum	Garden parsnip
	Heracleum mantegazzianum	Giant hogweed
	Heracleum sphondylium	Cow parsnip
	Heracleum laciniatum	Tromso palm
	Pastinaca sativa	Wild parsnip
	Peucedanum oreoselium	Mountain parsley
	Peucedanum ostruthium	Masterwort
Rutaceae	*Ruta graveolens*	Common rue
	Citrus bergamia	Bergamot lime
	Citrus aurantifolia	Persian lime
	Citrus aurantium	Lime
	Dictamnus alba	Gas plant
	Peucedanum galbanum	Blister bush
Moraceae	*Ficus carica*	Fig

Mechanism of phototoxicity

The phototoxicity associated with linear psoralens involves penetration of the chemical into keratinocytes/lymphocytes and other skin cells producing a two photon-dependent DNA cross-linking process (141), the presence and repair of which may result in apoptosis or accumulation of mutations. In the case of PUVA (psoralen + UVA photochemotherapy), repeated mild phototoxicity can be turned to therapeutic benefit to treat psoriasis, dermatitis, and other inflammatory dermatoses.

In the case of plant exposure, typically the course, of erythema/ blistering follows a delayed course, often with a gap of 24–96 hours after light exposure before maximum skin effect occurs. This makes diagnosis difficult where the causal event has been forgotten. On occasions, delayed presentation at A&E departments can be misdiagnosed as child abuse with alarming consequences.

Another chemical, hypericin, which is present in St John's wort, produces a similar problem as the psoralen family but by a different mechanism.

Clinical phytophotodermatitis features depend upon the "at risk" occupations (gardening, farming, canning, and cooking). Despite the advent of indoor pursuits such as computer games, phytophotodermatitis continues to present in children playing with plants out of doors during the summer holidays. Perhaps the commonest modern problem seen in adults relates to rotary mower or strimmer use (142) where unprotected exposed skin is splattered with psoralen-containing sap from such plants as cow parsley/parsnip thrown up by these mechanical devices. Subsequent sufficient doses of UVA exposure in sunlight produces characteristic acute (143) and chronic effects (144).

Selective breeding of celery designed to increase the shelf-life for retail purposes has resulted in higher concentrations of psoralen than seen previously. Enhancement of psoralen content is also seen if celery undergoes a fungal attack; the celery cells respond by enhancing psoralen levels. Occasionally, kitchen cooks can get sufficient quantities of psoralen from celery, parsnips, limes, oranges, vegetables, or fruit punches into their skin that, if followed by sunlight or sunbed exposure (145), can produce a marked blistering phototoxic effect.

In a similar fashion, if enough parsnip or celery soup is ingested, it is possible to induce a cutaneous phototoxic reaction with psoralen gaining access by ingestion rather than the topical route. The most evident of psoralen-containing plants, often seen along the side of railway tracks or riverbanks, is the giant hogweed, *Heracleum mantegazzianum*, which originates from the Ural Mountain region in Russia (146). A brush with the plant sap produces typical linear lesions (147) most frequently seen in fishermen and bathers, followed by pigmentation (144); even more striking are perioral blisters in children who use the hollow stems as pea shooters.

Berloque dermatitis is a problem less commonly seen today from the removal or lowering of the concentration of a traditional plant psoralen containing extract oil of bergamot, which in the past was added to fragrances. This agent, which is sourced from the bergamot lime in Italy, contains 5-methoxypsoralen. Used as a mixing agent for fragrances, it produces a classic psoralen phototoxicity pendant pattern if applied to the skin prior to sunlight exposure.

Occasionally a heavy exposure to airborne Compositae (daisy family) material can have the appearance of phototoxicity. It is known that this family of plants contain phototoxins of a non-psoralen type (for example, alfa-terthenyl). It is not yet clear whether the clinical phenomenon is simply photo-aggravation of contact allergy to Compositae or a true phototoxic reaction in its own right.

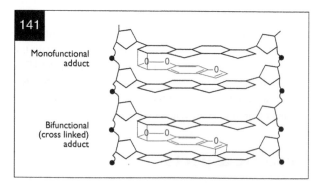

141

Monofunctional adduct

Bifunctional (cross linked) adduct

141: Cross-linking incorporation of psoralen between the two strands of DNA is initially formation of a monofunctional adduct. The damaging cross-link is completed by the energy of a second longer wavelength photon so producing the bifunctional adduct.

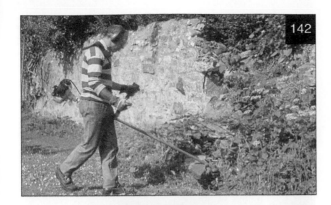

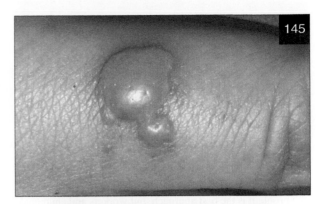

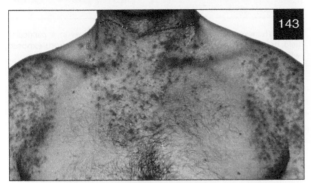

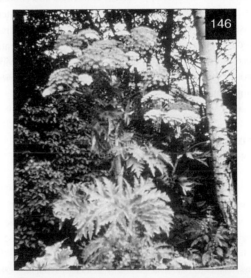

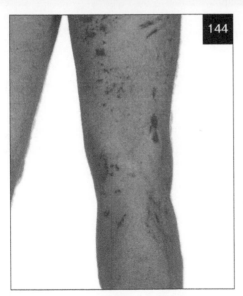

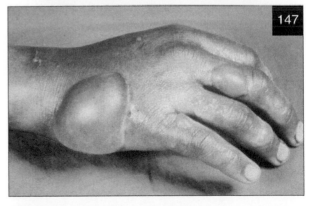

142: Although wearing face, hands and ear protectors, the person using the strimmer has exposed forearms and is currently working on a patch containing cow parsley/parsnip and would be expected to have psoralen-containing sap on his skin.

143: This vest-wearing gardener has developed the characteristic blistering lesions seen in strimmer's dermatitis 48 hours after strimming.

144: Three weeks after a blistering phototoxic response to cow parsley, this bather has developed characteristic chronic pigmentation.

145: This cook, who had been making celery soup, exposed her skin to a sunbed. Some 48 hours later, scattered blisters appeared on her hand and later became pigmented.

146: Giant hogweed often seen at the side of roads, railway tracks and streams.

147: Typical linear blistering on the hand of a child exposed to giant hogweed sap and to sunlight.

Phytophotodermatitis is not solely confined to the human species. Pigs and cattle are particularly prone to hypericin phototoxicity (St John's wort). Typically, a Friesian calf has phototoxic damage affecting the white patches on back and other photo-exposed areas. Often these can slough off as a result of the phototoxic burn, only to regrow later (**148**).

Treatment

Prevention of direct skin sap contact through awareness of the problem is the best approach, but workers and children do come in contact with the sap and sunlight. Large blisters, if necessary, can be burst with a sterile needle, antiseptic applied and patients warned that post-phototoxic pigmentation can persist for many months or even years. There is no evidence that potent topical steroid use in established phytophotodermatitis has any beneficial effect.

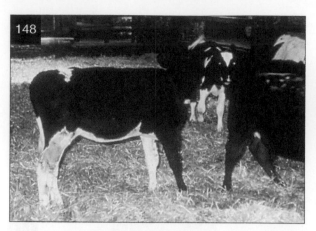

148: Whenever a farmer grazed young Friesian calves in a particular field, he noticed they tended to lose the skin from the photo-exposed white areas. St John's wort-associated phototoxicity was the culprit.

Reference

1. Klaber R. Phyto-photo-dermatitis. *Br J Dermatol* 1942;**54**:193–211.

Further reading

Gilchrest BA, Soter NA, Stoff JS, Mihm MC. The human sunburn reaction: histologic and biolchemical studies J Am Acad Dermatol 1981;**5**:411–22.

Hawk J. Photodermatology. London: Arnold, 1999.

Ortonne J, Marks R. Photodamaged Skin. Martin London: Dunitz, 1999.

Weedon D. Skin Pathology, 2nd Edn. London: Churchill Livingstone, 2002.

15 Photohistopathology
Graham Lowe

Photodermatoses

The microscopic appearances of the inflammatory photodermatoses are sometimes characteristic, but often non-specific. Close clinicopathologic correlation is required to optimize the chance of diagnostic success.

Chronic actinic dermatitis (CAD)

Biopsy specimens of involved skin show a spectrum of histopathologic appearances dependent on age and activity of the disease process. Mild disease will show a non-specific dermatitic appearance, with an upper dermal predominantly mononuclear infiltrate, exocytosis of inflammatory cells into variably spongiotic epidermis, focal parakeratosis, and mild acanthosis. This is also the appearance seen when lesions are induced by phototesting, simulating the picture of allergic contact dermatitis (149).

More severe disease leads to pronounced acanthosis with little spongiosis, along with dermal fibrosis, scattered stellate fibroblasts and vertical orientation of collagen fibers, similar to that seen in lichen simplex from persistent scratching, but in this case showing considerably more dermal inflammation (150). This inflammatory infiltrate may be band-like or diffuse, extending into the mid- and lower dermis, with a polymorphic phenotype consisting of lymphocytes (including hyperchromatic or convoluted forms resembling Sézary cells), plasma cells, eosinophils, giant cells, blast cells, and mitotic figures (151). The lymphoid cells may infiltrate the epidermis and mimic Pautrier micro-abscesses. The microscopic picture in this end of the pathologic spectrum simulates cutaneous T cell lymphoma, and is often referred to as actinic reticuloid.

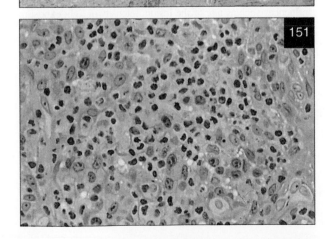

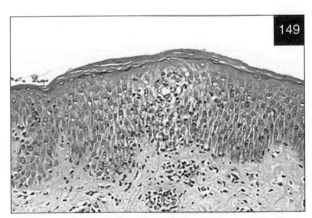

149: H+E. Chronic actinic dermatitis phototest site – non-specific dermatitis.
150: H+E thin section. Chronic actinic dermatitis – prominent acanthosis and upper/mid-dermal inflammation.
151: H+E thin section. Chronic actinic dermatitis – polymorphic inflammatory infiltrate.

This spectrum of appearances is similar to that encountered in contact dermatitis, where the severe pseudolymphomatous form may result from persistent antigenic stimulation.

The clinical and histologic resemblance to the following suggest that this condition has a delayed hypersensitivity pathogenesis:
- dermatitis
- induced lesions peaking at 24–48 hours
- predominant T cell phenotype
- CD4+ dominance except in cases with more florid histologic changes
- adhesion molecule expression similarity to tuberculin reactions, and
- allergic contact dermatitis, and clinical response to T cell immunomodulatory drugs.

Polymorphic light eruption

The clinical diversity of polymorphic light eruption is reflected in the variable histologic features encountered. An early lesion will show only a non-specific upper dermal perivascular inflammatory infiltrate, whereas a well-developed papular lesion will show characteristic superficial and deep perivascular accumulation of lymphocytes, accompanied by papillary dermal edema of variable degree. If the edema is prominent, then the infiltrate is often interstitial as well as perivascular (152). Occasionally, the degree of edema is such that the collagen connections are broken and subepidermal blister formation occurs (153).

The epidermis may appear normal, but spongiosis, which uncommonly can be severe enough to cause vesiculation simulating allergic dermatitis, may be present. Basal liquefaction is not infrequent (154), but cell death is an unusual feature.

These variable histologic features may reflect a number of influences such as age of the lesion, intensity of light exposure and individual sensitivity/immunologic reactivity.

Immunohistochemistry shows a T cell-dominated infiltrate, peaking at 72 hours, early appearance of CD4+ cells later giving way to CD8+ dominance, with increased numbers of dermal and epidermal Langerhans cells. This similarity to tuberculin reactions and allergic contact dermatitis, together with the pattern of adhesion molecule expression in evolving lesions, suggests that polymorphic light eruption also has a delayed hypersensitivity pathogenesis.

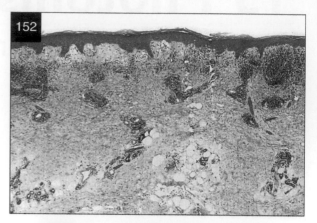

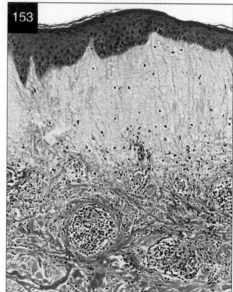

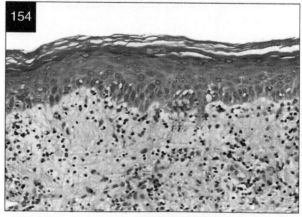

152: H+E. Polymorphic light eruption – well-established lesion with prominent inflammation and subepidermal edema.

153: H+E. Polymorphic light eruption – severe edema resulting in subepidermal blister formation

154: H+E Polymorphic light eruption – basal epidermal liquefaction.

Actinic prurigo

The histologic features may be similar to those seen in polymorphic light eruption, with predominantly lymphocytic perivascular inflammation around upper and mid-dermal vessels (**155**). The distinct HLA typing in actinic prurigo, however, suggests pathophysiologic differences between the two conditions.

Lymphoid follicles are sometimes present, particularly in cheilitis and conjunctivitis. Prurigenous areas will show excoriation and changes of lichen simplex.

Hydroa vacciniforme

Reticular degeneration leads to intra-epidermal vesiculation, with underlying predominantly lymphocytic perivascular inflammation and occasional hemorrhage (**156**). Subsequent necrosis and ulceration of the epidermis and subjacent dermis, which is accompanied by a mixed cellular infiltrate, will lead to variable scarring as the lesions heal (**157**).

Solar urticaria

As in other forms of urticaria, there is a superficial mixed cellular infiltrate, dilatation of small blood vessels and lymphatics, and dermal edema, recognized by separation of collagen bundles. Granulocytes appear within 5 minutes and increase in a dose-dependent manner up to 2 hours. Mast cells and eosinophils degranulate, the latter depositing eosinophil major basic protein. After 24 hours, mononuclear cells predominate. A few patients with more severe reactions show a leukocytoclastic picture, similar to that seen in urticarial vasculitis (**158**).

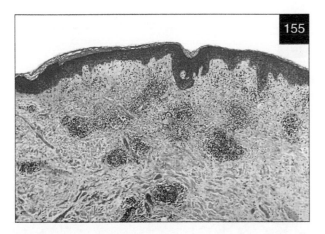

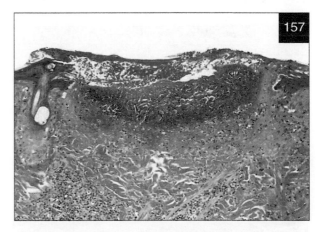

155: H+E. Actinic prurigo – resembling polymorphic light eruption with upper/mid-dermal inflammation and subepidermal edema.
156: H+E. Hydroa vacciniforme – reticular degeneration of the epidermis leading to vesiculation.

157: H+E. Hydroa vacciniforme – later lesion showing necrosis of epidermis and subjacent dermis.
158: H+E. Solar vasculitis – leuckocytoclastic vasculitis.

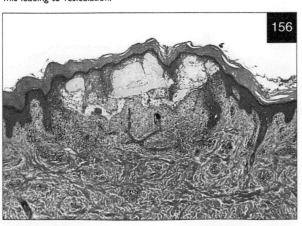

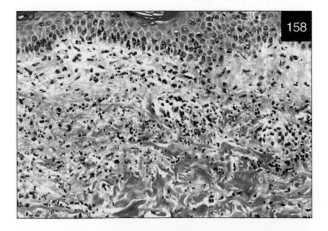

Porphyria and pseudoporphyria

The characteristic histologic feature in the cutaneous porphyrias is the deposition of PAS-positive diastase-resistant amorphous hyaline material in and around the walls of upper dermal blood vessels, and often at the dermo-epidermal junction (**159**). This represents excessively synthesized basement membrane material resulting from repetitive cycles of damage and repair. It is most prominent in erythropoietic protoporphyria, where perivascular deposits of leaked serum components contribute to irregular cuffing around the vessels.

Clinical blisters are subepidermal, resulting from splitting in the lamina lucida, with the PAS-positive basement membrane usually found in the roof of the blister. Projection of the dermal papillae into the floor of the blister (festooning) is common, and the inflammatory infiltrate typically sparse (**160**).

In the bullous, presumed phototoxic reaction, pseudoporphyria, blisters are also subepidermal, although festooning is not always prominent, and hyaline material is not usually present in early lesions. The inflammatory infiltrate may contain an occasional eosinophil.

Drug photosensitivity

Clinically, phototoxic reactions often resemble an exaggerated sunburn reaction, the microscopic appearance varying from apoptotic "sunburn cells" to epidermal necrosis, with mild underlying inflammation (**161**).

Photo-allergic reactions may resemble contact allergic dermatitis, with spongiotic vesiculation in severe cases (**162**), or may show a lichenoid tissue reaction. The same drug can cause a range of clinical and histologic appearances.

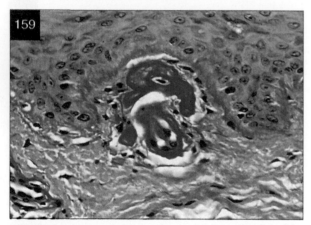

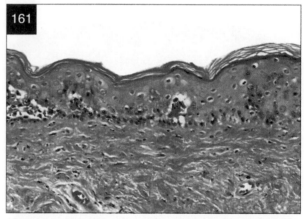

159: PAS. Porphyria – deposition of PAS-positive material in upper dermal blood vessels.
160: H+E. Porphyria cutanea tarda – cell-poor subepidermal blister with festooning of dermal papillae.

161: H+E. Phototoxic reaction – "sunburn cells" and little inflammation.
162: H+E. Photoallergic reaction – spongiotic vesiculation.

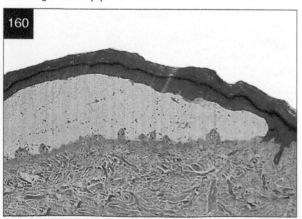

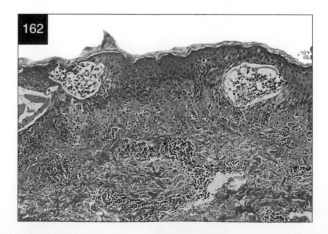

Photodamage

Sunburn

The characteristic histologic feature of acute ultraviolet damage to the skin is damaged keratinocytes known as "sunburn cells", caused by UVB. On hematoxylin and eosin stained sections, these typically have a shrunken dark (blue) pyknotic nucleus with dense eosinophilic (red) cytoplasm (**163**). Lesser degrees of damage may show cytoplasmic vacuolation, nuclear swelling or "cloudy" cytoplasmic swelling.

Sunburn cells appear as early as 30 minutes after irradiation. They are maximal at 24 hours, when they are distributed throughout the epidermis. By 72 hours, they are mainly confined to the superficial layers. These cells have sustained significant DNA damage, retain a basal-cell level of differentiation immunohistochemically, and are being eliminated by a process termed apoptosis.

Langerhans cells become depleted within 24 hours, and take 2–3 weeks to return to baseline. Other features include spongiosis, mast cell depletion/degranulation, early neutrophil infiltration, and endothelial cell enlargement within the superficial vascular plexus.

Solar elastosis

This is the histologic hallmark of chronic ultraviolet radiation damage. Separated from the epidermis by a narrow band of normal-appearing collagen (Grenz zone) is connective tissue that stains a bluer color than normal in hematoxylin and eosin preparations, so-called basophilic degeneration of collagen (**164**). This tissue exhibits the tinctorial staining properties of elastic fibers, and is often referred to as elastotic material or solar elastosis (**165**).

This damaged tissue appears initially as thickened interwoven fibers in the upper dermis, but with increasing severity becomes more amorphous and extensive, and may stain less strongly. Histologic evidence of solar elastosis predates clinical signs of photodamage, and is often observed in early adulthood. Biochemically, this tissue is elastin, although disorganized and with abnormal constituent proportions. Its origin has been the subject of much debate. Degradation of collagen and/or elastic fibers and actinic stimulation of fibroblasts have been proposed. The low-grade accompanying inflammatory component may be of fundamental importance.

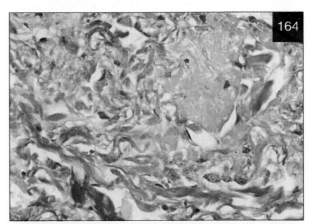

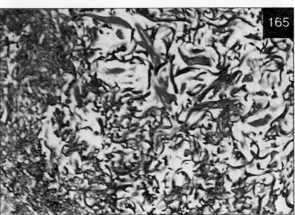

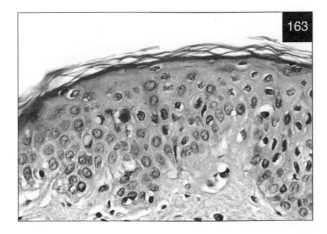

163: H+E. Sunburn – typical apoptotic "sunburn cells" at different stages of evolution.
164: H+E. Solar elastosis – basophilic (bluish) discoloration of affected connective tissue.
165: EVG. Solar elastosis – few remaining collagen fibers (red) amongst elastotic tissue.

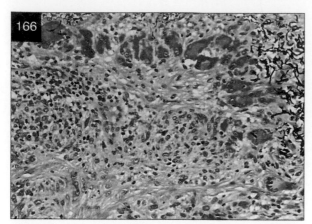

166: ERY. Actinic granuloma – giant cells and elastoclasis at rim of lesion.

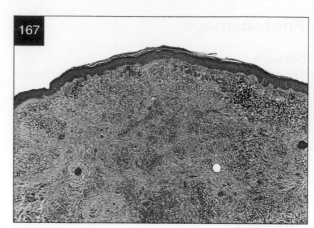

167: ERY. Actinic granuloma – loss of elastic tissue and fibrosis within central zone.

Actinic granuloma (O'Brien)

The rim of annular lesions shows dermal infiltration by mononuclear and foreign body giant cells, the latter engulfing elastotic fibers – known as elastoclasis (166). Within the central zone there is loss of elastic and elastotic fibers, with some fibrosis (167). Necrobiosis is not a feature. A cell-mediated immune response to elastotic fibers has been postulated.

Further reading

Gilchrest BA, Soter NA, Stoff JS, Mihm MC. The human sunburn reaction: histologic and biochemical studies. *J Am Acad Dermatol* 1981;**5**:411–22.

Hawk J. *Photodermatology*. London: Arnold, 1999.

Ortonne J, Marks R. *Photodamaged Skin*. London: Martin Dunitz, 1999.

Weedon D. *Skin Pathology, 2nd edn*. London: Churchill Livingstone, 2002.

16 Porphyrin Biochemistry: Laboratory Studies

Julie Woods

Porphyrins are tetracyclic molecules (**168**) named for the Greek word for purple *(porphuros)*. Because of their delocalized electronic structure porphyrins can shuttle electrons around and chelate metal ions. This makes them the principal molecules of energy capture and transfer. As such, porphyrin-containing proteins are involved in diverse and fundamental biochemical processes such as oxygen transport (hemoglobin), light capture (chlorophyll), antioxidant defense (catalase), and xenobiotic metabolism (P450 enzymes). The porphyrins are found as metal ion-bound prosthetic groups within these key enzymes, and mediate the transfer of electrons during the metabolic reactions that are catalyzed by them. The two most important prosthetic groups are heme (iron-chelated porphyrin) and chlorophyll (magnesium-chelated porphyrin). In fact the heme prosthetic group is so fundamental to life that its biosynthesis is one of the most highly conserved biochemical pathways.

Heme synthesis

In humans, primarily the liver and bone marrow synthesize porphyrins, but almost every cell possesses the capability to make them. Most of our knowledge comes from study of the heme biosynthesis in the liver. However, regulation of biosynthesis is likely to differ between tissue types because of the different demands for heme-containing proteins. The actual precursors involved in the heme biosynthetic pathway are the colorless porphyrinogens, which are unstable and readily convert to the conjugated, highly colored porphyrins on exposure to light and oxygen. As porphyrins are such chemically reactive molecules their production is kept under efficient control. It has been estimated that less than 2% of precursors required for heme synthesis are produced in excess.

Porphyrin synthesis begins in the mitochondria with the synthesis of delta-aminolevulinic acid (ALA) from glycine and succinyl CoA. ALA synthetase, which catalyzes the reaction, is probably the most important rate-limiting enzyme in the pathway, a detail exploited by ALA-photodynamic therapy. In the cytoplasm, two ALA molecules then condense to form the monopyrrole porphobilinogen (PBG). PBG condenses to form hydroxymethylbilane, which is then converted to uroporphyrinogen. Uroporphyrinogen is then gradually decarboxylated,

168: The structures of uroporphyrin, coproporphyrin and protoporphyrin. Note the number of carboxyl groups on each molecule; uroporphyrin has eight, coproporphyrin has four and protoporphyrin has two.

ultimately forming protoporphyrin, which is localized in the mitochondria for insertion of an iron atom by the enzyme ferrochelatase (**169**).

Porphyria

Sometimes heme biosynthesis can go wrong, resulting in a build-up of porphyrins in body fluids and tissues as the unstable porphyrinogens auto-oxidize. Because the liver and erythropoietic tissues synthesize the bulk of the body's porphyrins, overproduction usually occurs in these tissues.

As a consequence the excess porphyrins spill over into the bile, blood, and urine. Porphyrin overproduction usually occurs from a decrease in activity in one of the enzymes responsible for porphyrin biosynthesis, and the resulting group of disorders are known as the porphyrias. There are at least seven distinct porphyrias, each arising from one of the enzymes of the biosynthetic pathway *(Table 16.1)*. The underlying molecular cause responsible for the decrease in activity is usually a defect in the gene encoding the enzyme; however, porphyria cutanea tarda (PCT) can also be acquired as a result of lifestyle factors and this acquired form accounts for about 80% of cases. Porphyrias can be subdivided depending on whether there is cutaneous involvement or on the basis of their tissue of origin. Neurovisceral symptoms are attributed to an excess of porphyrin precursors (ALA and PBG) and acute deficiency of heme in the liver, whereas an excess of porphyrins causes skin photosensitivity, blistering, and erosion. The photodependent changes caused by porphyrin accumulation in the skin (**170**) occur because porphyrins are very powerful photosensitizers. Almost all the cutaneous symptoms of porphyria

169: The heme biosynthetic pathway.

Table 16.1: **Listing of the main forms of porphyria**

Porphyria	Enzyme affected	Cutaneous involvement	Chromosome location	Inheritance
ALA dehydratase deficiency porphyria (plumboporphyria)	ALA dehydratase	No	9q34	Recessive
Acute intermittent porphyria (AIP)	Porphobilinogen deaminase	No	11q24.1-11q24.2	Dominant
Congenital erythropoietic porphyria (CEP) (Günther disease)	Uroporphyrinogen III synthase	Yes	10q25.2-10q26.3	Recessive
Porphyria cutanea tarda (PCT)	Uroporphyrinogen decarboxylase	Yes	1p34 (≈10%)	Dominant
Hepatoerythropoietic porphyria (HEP)	Uroporphyrinogen decarboxylase	Yes	(Homozygous variant of PCT)	Recessive
Hereditary coproporphyria (CP)	Coproporphyrinogen oxidase	Yes	3q12	Dominant
Variegate porphyria (VP)	Protoporphyrinogen oxidase	Yes	1q21-1q23	Dominant
Erythropoietic protoporphyria (EPP)	Ferrochelatase	Yes	18q21.3	Dominant

are caused by a waveband of 400–415 nm, which is located within the so-called Soret band (**171**). The delocalized electrons of porphyrins absorb light in this region and become elevated from the ground state to the excited singlet state. The excited molecule can either return to ground state, releasing the energy as heat and light (**172**), or convert to the excited triplet state via intersystem crossing (**173**). In the presence of oxygen, the excited triplet state can result in the production of singlet oxygen and other reactive oxygen species, which damage cells. Uroporphyrin and coproporphyrin are relatively water soluble and can diffuse out of the capillaries into the epidermis. Protoporphyrin is the least water soluble and stays within the blood vessel. This discrepancy in the localization of the chromophores may partly explain the different cutaneous symptoms seen in variegate porphyria (VP), PCT, and erythropoietic protoporphyria (EPP) on exposure to light.

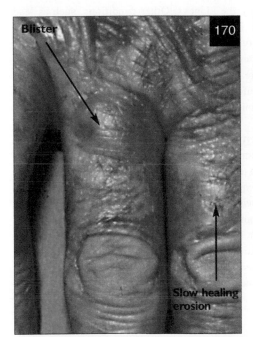

170: Photo-induced skin changes in the hand of a patient with PCT. Note the blister and erosion (arrowed).

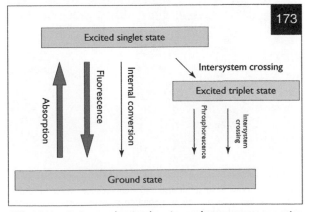

172: Porphyrins, such as protoporphyrin, absorb blue light in the Soret region, and emit the energy in the form of light of a longer wavelength, hence the red fluorescence of porphyrins.

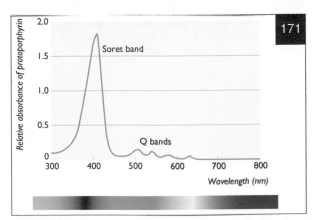

171: Absorbance spectrum of protoporphyrin showing the Soret band and Q bands.

173: A Jablonski diagram showing the primary photoprocesses occurring between electronic states of molecules.

Biochemical porphyria testing as part of the photosensitivity investigation

Background

In photodermatology the goal of biochemical porphyrin investigation is to determine whether cutaneous photosensitivity, blistering and so on are due to abnormally elevated levels of porphyrins in body fluids and tissues, and to provide a diagnosis of the specific porphyria involved. Once diagnosed, biochemistry is then used subsequently to aid management of the porphyric patient; for example, plasma fluorimetry can be used to monitor the patient with PCT as clinical symptoms will disappear as the porphyrin levels in the blood decline. However, it is important to remember that there is no single test that can account for all possibilities in porphyria, and consequently the array of tests can seem confusing.

The different porphyrias are characterized by particular patterns of overproduction of porphyrins and/or their precursors. Porphyrins can be separated on the basis of their chemical properties as they differ in polarity and acid solubility because of the number of carboxyl groups (protoporphyrin is less water soluble than uroporphyrin, which is why the former is more likely to be detected in the feces as a result of excretion via the bile, and the latter is found in urine and plasma). They can be detected because they absorb blue light and emit this energy in the form of red light (**174**). For the purposes of this chapter we will be concerned only with the detection of porphyria with skin involvement. Biochemical tests for porphyrin precursors, the diagnosis of AIP or acute attacks of porphyria will not be discussed.

Other conditions

Drugs such as naproxen and tetracycline can provoke the clinical features of PCT. However, no biochemical markers of true porphyria (that is, abnormally raised porphyrin levels) are found, and so this condition is often referred to as pseudoporphyria. There is also a pseudoporphyria of renal failure, where porphyrin levels accumulate from decreased clearance by the kidneys. Other conditions, such as lead poisoning, iron deficiency anemia, excessive alcohol consumption, gastrointestinal bleeding, and hepatitis C infection, can result in elevated porphyrins being detected by one or more of the tests. This highlights the importance of gathering information from a battery of tests in conjunction with the clinical symptoms.

Equipment

Although empiric observations of porphyrin fluorescence in body fluids can be made using a Wood's lamp, in reality specialized equipment is necessary for the accurate measurement and identification of porphyrins. The most useful instruments for the diagnosis of cutaneous porphyrias are the spectrophotometer, spectrofluorimeter (**175**) and HPLC. It is recommended that equipment with fluorescence detection be fitted with a red-sensitive photomultiplier to increase sensitivity. The fluorimeter should be calibrated using commercially

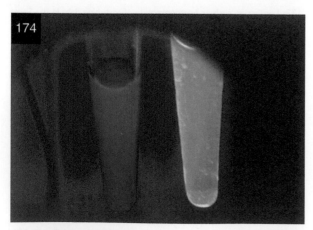

174: Porphyrins exhibit intense red fluorescence when irradiated with blue light. On the left is a solution of protoporphyrin, on the right is a control solution.

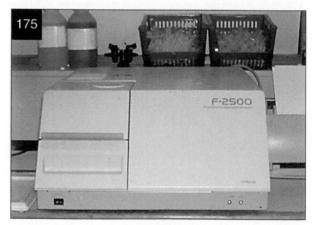

175: The fluorescence spectrophotometer. This instrument is the workhorse of the porphyrin biochemistry laboratory.

available porphyrin standards. Additional equipment includes a microwave, balance, and glass microscope slides for weighing and drying fecal samples, centrifuges adapted to process clinical samples, and a fume cupboard. A preparation area with appropriate adjustable lighting and adequate measures in place for the handling, disposal and spillage of potentially high-risk samples is necessary. All of the sample preparation can be performed in sterile, disposable plastic vessels such as microcentrifuge tubes, 30 ml universal containers, or disposable soda glass tubes, with the exception of the fecal analysis, which requires heavy-walled glass test tubes. Chemicals required include ethyl acetate, acetic acid, diethyl ether, ethanol, and phosphate-buffered saline (**176**). Most of the quantitative/semiquantitative methods of porphyrin analysis involve adding hydrochloric acid to the samples, which helps to convert the colorless porphyrinogens to porphyrins and enhance light absorption. Calibration standards and quality control materials can be purchased or in the latter case prepared by the laboratory if there is no commercially available material. Reference ranges should be determined using standard methods.

Sample collection

Porphyrins, particularly protoporphyrin, are extremely labile when exposed to light; consequently the samples must be wrapped in tinfoil and protected from light during collection, transport, storage, and analysis. There is an association between PCT and hepatitis infection, so all suspected PCT cases should be treated as high risk.

Blood

Venous blood is collected into EDTA-containing blood tubes. If samples are to be forwarded to an external testing laboratory for screening, then the blood should be centrifuged at low speed to pellet the cells and the plasma decanted to a separate container (**177**). The plasma and cell pellet can then be sent in the post in an appropriate container for clinical sample transport.

Urine

It is now generally accepted that 24-hour urine collections are not necessary for porphyrin analysis, and that a fresh, random (preferably early morning) sample of about 20 ml is sufficient. The level of urine creatinine must be determined for each sample. Those that fall below 4 mmol/liter should be rejected as being too dilute for accurate analysis and a further sample obtained. The collecting tubes must be wrapped in tinfoil, kept cool and protected from light at all times.

Feces

About 5–10 g of a fresh fecal sample is required for analysis. The sample should be protected from light, and kept cool or frozen during transport.

Biochemical investigation of blood
Qualitative plasma fluorimetry

Plasma fluorimetry is a rapid screening test that will detect cutaneous porphyria provided the patient is in the symptomatic phase. Elevated levels of plasma porphyrin are found in patients with symptoms of PCT, EPP, VP, HC, and CEP.

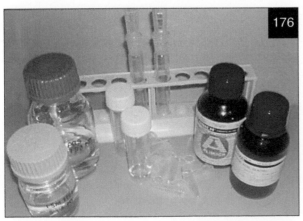

176: In recent years the methods used to extract and quantitate porphyrins from body fluids have been transformed. This figure illustrates the types of glassware, plastics, and chemicals used in the analytic process.

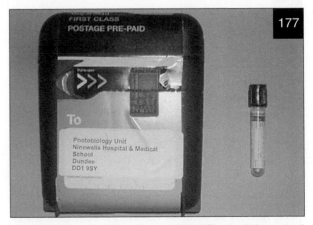

177: A sample bottle for the collection of blood. This should be wrapped in tinfoil to protect it from light, and appropriately labeled. Also shown is a typical transport container made of rigid plastic and sealed. This protects both the sample from breakage, and also personnel (for example, postal workers) from any possible risk of contamination.

Technically the test is straightforward. Plasma is diluted with phosphate-buffered saline and the samples placed in the fluorimeter. The fluorescence emission (550–700 nm) is measured at an excitation wavelength of 400 nm (**178**). Abnormally raised plasma porphyrins are identified as a characteristic peak in the emission spectrum *(Table 16.2)*. Some typical emission scans obtained from normal subjects and patients with active PCT, EPP, and VP are shown in **179**. This screening test is therefore mainly used to imply or exclude a cutaneous porphyria diagnosis in symptomatic patients. If no peak is detected then photosensitization by porphyrins can be excluded as a cause of the active skin lesions. If the scan is positive then further testing should always follow. A retrospective study of plasma scan results obtained at Ninewells Hospital over a 5-year period estimated the sensitivity (100% [95% CI 95–100%]) and specificity (99% [95% CI 98.4–99.6%]) of a positive plasma scan as a diagnostic test.

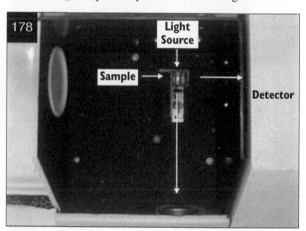

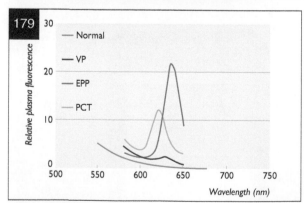

178: An interior view of the spectrophotofluorimeter looking down from the top. The sample is in place and is being irradiated with 405 nm (violet) light. Note the intense red fluorescence of the sample. A detector is situated at right angles to the light path, to collect the emitted red fluorescence.

179: Plasma emission spectrofluorimetry. Some typical emission scans obtained from normal subjects and patients with active PCT, EPP, and VP. The peak maxima are shown in *Table 16.2*.

Quantitative determination of porphyrin levels in blood
The total erythrocyte porphyrin test allows the quantification of porphyrins from erythrocytes. Erythrocyte porphyrins are elevated in patients with EPP, CEP and occasionally in VP and HC. In addition to porphyria, there are several other conditions that result in an increase in erythrocyte porphyrins, including iron deficiency anemia, hemolytic anemia and lead poisoning. However, in these latter disorders the elevated species is usually zinc-chelated protoporphyrin, which is not phototoxic and can be distinguished from the free protoporphyrin that predominates in EPP (see below).

The test as described measures total erythrocyte porphyrins, as the analytic conditions convert zinc-chelated protoporphyrin to free protoporphyrin.[1] The method used for quantification involves extracting the erythrocyte porphyrins into freshly prepared ethyl acetate/acetic acid (3:1, v/v), then transferring them to 1.5 mol/liter hydrochloric acid. The fluorescence emission is measured between 550 and 700 nm at an excitation wavelength of 405 nm. The fluorescence of the extracted porphyrins (mainly protoporphyrin) is compared to a standard solution of coproporphyrin and an adjustment made to account for the difference in the fluorescence intensities of protoporphyrin and coproporphyrin. In a more recent modification of this method, whole blood is diluted with phosphate-buffered saline and extracted into freshly prepared diethyl ether:acetic acid (4:1 v/v). The porphyrins are then transferred to 2.7 M hydrochloric acid. With the emission wavelength set at 602 nm, the excitation spectrum is recorded between 350 nm and 450 nm. The fluorescence of the samples is compared with the fluorescence of a uroporphyrin standard solution.

Table 16.2: **Table of expected plasma flourescence emission maxima**

Porphyria	Plasma	Emission maxima (nm)
PCT	Uroporphyrin	619–621
HC	Coproporphyrin	619–621
CEP	Coproporphyrin/uroporphyrin/protoporphyrin	619–621
EPP	Protoporphyrin	634–636
VP	Coproporphyrin/protoporphyrin	626

Qualitative whole blood fluorimetry

To distinguish EPP from the other porphyrias and conditions that result in an abnormal increase in erythrocyte porphyrins, the relative amounts of free, unchelated protoporphyrin and zinc-chelated protoporphyrin (Zn-protoporphyrin) should be determined. Because the acid extraction procedure of the total erythrocyte porphyrin test strips the zinc moiety from zinc-chelated protoporphyrin, a procedure is used where erythrocyte porphyrins are extracted under neutral conditions using ethanol, allowing discrimination between zinc-chelated protoporphyrin (Zn-protoporphyrin) and unchelated free protoporphyrin. Briefly, whole blood is diluted in phosphate-buffered saline and then extracted with 95% ethanol (v/v). The fluorescence emission spectrum of the ethanolic supernatant is determined at an excitation wavelength of 415 nm. A major peak at 590–591 nm in the emission spectrum suggests the predominance of Zn-protoporphyrin; a major peak at 633–634 nm suggests the predominance of free protoporphyrin. In normal subjects the 590–591 nm peak predominates, which excludes EPP. If the major peak is found at 633–634 nm, then this confirms the diagnosis of EPP (**180**).

Fluorescing erythrocytes: "fluorocytes"

Erythrocyte porphyrins abnormally raised as a result of EPP and CEP can also be detected microscopically. Fresh blood is diluted in saline and placed on a microscope slide. When viewed under UV light, approximately 10–30% of the erythrocytes will fluoresce brightly (fluorocytes; **181**). The fluorescence rapidly fades (within seconds) and is rarely seen in blood from normal subjects. More persistent fluorescence is observed in erythrocytes from patients with CEP. Fluorescent erythrocytes have also been studied by flow cytometry, which may be a way to quantify this method. This assessment is rarely used as a front-line test to diagnose porphyria, but it may be a useful supplementary tool.

Biochemical investigation of urine and feces

Urine is added to 0.27 M hydrochloric acid and the fluorescence emission is measured at 596 nm at an excitation wavelength of 350–450 nm. The fluorescence is then compared against that of a solution of coproporphyrin of known concentration and results expressed as moles of porphyrin per millimole of creatinine. Patients with symptomatic PCT, HC, CEP, and VP will have abnormally elevated levels of urinary porphyrins. Other conditions that result in an increase in urinary porphyrins include liver failure and lead poisoning.

Fecal porphyrins are raised in PCT, HC, VP, CEP, and occasionally EPP. Other conditions that influence fecal porphyrin excretion include gastrointestinal bleeding and diet, particularly ones rich in red meat. Unlike the preceding methods, fecal analysis involves the spectrophotometer as opposed to the fluorescence spectrophotometer. A small amount of sample is dried and weighed prior to analysis. The remainder is homogenized in hydrochloric acid, and then extracted with ether. By adding water, compounds that might interfere with the test such as absorbing derivatives of chlorophyll and carotenoids, are trapped in the ether phase. The more hydrophilic phase is removed and scanned in a spectrophotometer. The concentration of total porphyrins is then calculated from the height of the Soret maxima and expressed as moles of porphyrin per gram of feces.

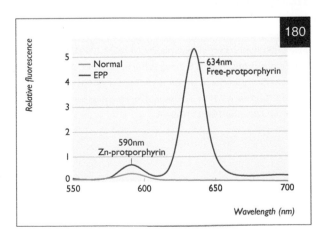

180: Fluorescence emission of free and zinc-chelated protoporphyrin. In patients with EPP, free protoporphyrin is greatly elevated.

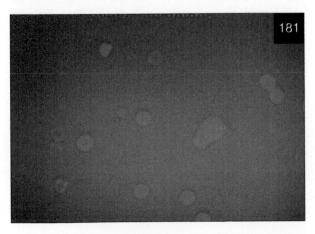

181: "Fluorocytes", or fluorescing erythrocytes, isolated from a patient with EPP. Normal erythrocytes do not fluoresce.

Table 16.3: **Table of diagnostic findings for laboratory testing of porphyrias**

Porphyria	Plasma	Erythrocytes	Urine	Faeces
PCT	Uroporphyrin	Normal	Uroporphyrin I Uroporphyrin III	Isocoproporphyrin
EPP	Protorphyrin	Free Protoporphyrin	Normal	Protoporphyrin normal
VP	Coproporphyrin Protorphyrin	Normal	Coproporphyrin III	Protoporphyrin Coproporphyrin III
HC	Coproporphyrin	Normal Slight increase	Coproporphyrin III	Coproporphyrin III
CEP	Uroporphyrin I Coproporphyrin I Protoporphyrin	Uroporphyrin I Coproporphyrin I Zn-protoporphyrin	Uroporphyrin I Coproporphyrin I	Coproporphyrin I

Definitive diagnosis

Definitive diagnosis of porphyria is achieved by characterizing the profile of porphyrins and precursors in the acidified urine and fecal extracts by HPLC. This will, for example, distinguish PCT from drug-induced pseudoporphyria (as would plasma screening) or HC (which plasma screening would not), or cases where the total amount of porphyrins may not be increased, but the excretion pattern has altered. For example, PCT patients can have distinct changes in urinary porphyrin profiles when in remission, although the total amount of urinary porphyrins falls within the normal range. An overview of typical biochemical findings following investigation of the different porphyrias is shown in *Table 16.3*. Thus, if plasma emission fluorimetry identifies an emission peak at ≈621 nm, then urine, fecal, and erythrocyte analysis should be performed to distinguish between PCT, HC, and CEP, whereas if the peak is centered around 636 nm, then erythrocyte porphyrins should be quantitated and the Zn-protoporphyrin:free protoporphyrin ratio determined to confirm or exclude a diagnosis of EPP.

Reference

1. Labbe RF, Vreman HJ, Stevenson DK. Zinc protoporphyrin: a metabolite with a mission. *Clin Chem* 1999;**45**:2060–72.

Further reading

Deacon AC, Elder GH. ACP Best Practice No 165: front line tests for the investigation of suspected porphyria. *J Clin Pathol* 2001;**54**:500–7.

Elder GH, Smith SG, Smyth SJ. Laboratory investigation of the porphyrias. *Ann Clin Biochem* 1990;**27**:395–412.

Gibbs NK, Traynor N, Ferguson J. Biochemical diagnosis of the cutaneous porphyrias: five years experience of plasma spectrofluorimetry. *Br J Dermatol* 1995;**133** (Suppl. 45):18.

Lockwood WH, Poulos V, Rossi E Curnow DH. Rapid procedure for fecal porphyrin assay. *Clin Chem* 1985;**31**:1163–7.

Moore MR. Biochemistry of porphyria. *Int J Biochem* 1993;**25**:1353–68.

Poh-Fitzpatrick MB, Piomelli S, Young P, Hsu H, Harber LC. Rapid quantitative assay for erythrocyte porphyrins. *Arch Dermatol* 1974;**110**:225–30.

Poulos V, Lockwood WH. A rapid method for estimating red blood cell porphyrin. *Int J Biochem* 1980;**12**:1049–50.

17 The Genophotodermatoses

James Ferguson

This rare group of inherited skin disorders is characterized by photosensitivity and a range of other clinical signs. The diagnosis is made on a combination of clinical features and laboratory investigations. These diseases, with the exception of Smith–Lemli–Opitz syndrome, are all due to genetic defects in the DNA repair processes.

DNA is continually subjected to both exogenous and endogenous mutagenesis.[1] Cells have evolved complex mechanisms to minimize mutations in actively transcribed genes. "Repair" of a mutation should occur before DNA replication when such mutations can become permanent in daughter cells. Important repair enzyme systems, such as specific base change repair, nucleotide excision repair (NER),[2] recombination repair, and postreplication repair, have defects that are associated with disease. Successful DNA repair is also dependent on the presentation of the DNA following DNA unzipping by enzymes of the helicase group.[3]

Nucleotide excision repair (NER)

NER is a type of DNA repair pathway which is highly conserved and found throughout living cells. The loss of this repair

Table 17.1: The genophotodermatoses

Condition	Defect
Xeroderma pigmentosum	Nucleotide excision repair
Cockayne syndrome	Nucleotide excision repair
Trichothiodystrophy	Nucleotide excision repair
Rothmund Thomson syndrome	DNA helicase
Bloom syndrome	DNA helicase
Smith–Lemli–Opitz syndrome	Cholesterol synthesis

activity gives rise to the clinical manifestations of xeroderma pigmentosum, Cockayne syndrome, and trichothiodystrophy.[2]

Xeroderma pigmentosum XP (classic type)

This rare, autosomal recessive disease, which affects both sexes equally, occurs in the European and North American populations at an incidence of 1:250,000. It is probably six times more common in North Africa and Japan.

In 1968, Cleaver discovered that some patients shown to have the disease, had a deficiency in excision repair of ultraviolet-induced DNA damage.[4]

Clinical manifestations

It has been known for some time that the clinical manifestations of this disease vary greatly between patients. All seem to suffer to some degree from dry skin and marked freckling of sunlight-exposed skin sites as well as an increased susceptibility to cutaneous malignancy seen even as early as 5 years of age. Other patients in addition experience severe ocular and neurologic problems leading to a reduced lifespan.

The key to understanding the origin of such clinical diversity has emerged from scientific laboratory study of the genetic heterogeneity of nucleotide excision repair. Specific grouping of defects following cell fusion techniques with fibroblast cell lines from other XP patients has recognized the ability to cancel out the defect. This has created the concept of complementation groups. From such work, a range of defects have emerged: specifically complementation groups A, B, D, and G are associated with neurologic defects owing primarily to neuronal degradation, the exact mechanism of which is unknown.

At birth the skin appears normal, for it requires the mutagenic effect of ultraviolet to produce the increased freckling, dryness, and hyperpigmentation of sunlight-exposed sites so characteristic of this disease (**182**). Another early feature is awareness of the severe sunburn response, which may be of delayed onset and persistent in duration. Such reactions can occur at much lower levels of sunlight exposure than seen in normal children (**183, 184**). This susceptibility continues on into later life.

Those severely affected begin to show the emergence of premalignant and malignant skin lesions in the first few years of life. Basal cell carcinomas (BCCs), squamous cell carcinomas (SCCs), and malignant melanomas are all seen; the latter (as in the normal population) can be fatal. Ophthalmic problems are also an important aspect of XP. These include photophobia, keratitis, xerosis, corneal opacification, and pterygium formation (**185**). Some patients with complementation group A have particularly severe neurologic signs. This is termed the De Sanctis–Cacchione syndrome,[5] where the cutaneous signs are accompanied by severe mental retardation, ataxia, spasticity, deafness, and hypogonadism.

Investigations

Monochromator or broadband UVB sources reveal erythema responses, which occur at lower doses than expected in normal subjects, and may be delayed in onset and persistent in duration. Certainty of the diagnosis of XP of either classic or variant types requires cell mutation study. This is still based on

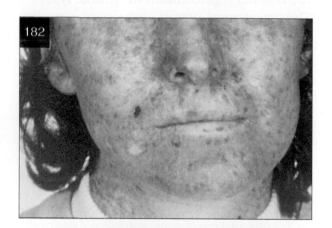

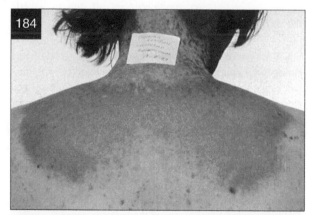

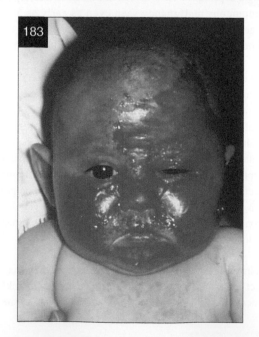

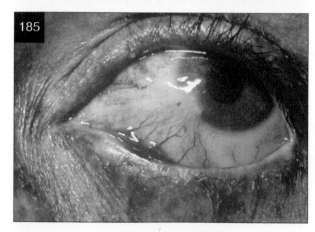

182: Freckling, depigmentation and scarring at the sites of tumor removal, characteristic of chronic changes seen in XP.

183: Acute photosensitivity seen as the first sign of XP in this infant following minimal sunlight exposure.

184: Sunburn following sunlight exposure while wearing a low-cut dress in a patient with classic XP.

185: Pterygium formation in a patient with XP. Note the partial loss of lower eyelashes.

fibroblast culture work and in the case of classic XP shows cells to be abnormally sensitive to UV, with a marked reduction in excision repair. Such study needs to be conducted in a specialist unit. The main differential diagnoses include those young patients with skin type 1 and freckles, as well as other members of the genophotodermatoses group.

Management

Management of patients is focused on early diagnosis and the careful protection of patients from the mutagenic effects of sunlight and other ultraviolet sources. Cancer surveillance and support for those patients with extracutaneous involvement is needed as appropriate. The true causal action spectrum for melanoma is still unknown. Many workers believe there is a role for UVA. Accordingly, avoidance of the whole UV spectrum is advisable. Careful use of photoprotective measures at school and at home is vital. Dermaguard, a sticky-backed plastic film, placed on car, house, and school windows can help to keep childhood as normal an experience as possible (see Chapter 4). It is important to assist parents by communicating directly with schools. Considerable help in this area can be obtained from the xeroderma pigmentosum website (http://www.xpsupportgroup.org.uk). Evidence does exist to support the view that today fewer XP patients are dying from their tumors. Mortality is more likely to occur as the result of neurologic/immune deficiency complications. Surveillance for malignancy is essential as is frequent follow-up and advice on the use of a broad-spectrum sun barrier.

Variant xeroderma pigmentosum (XPV)

This form of xeroderma pigmentosum may present in the second, third, or later decades. As with the classic form, it is rare, also inherited as autosomal recessive. It affects both sexes and is the diagnosis in about one-third of all XP cases. Unlike the classic type, delayed onset/severe photosensitivity is not a feature. Tumors do occur but much later. Neurologic features are not an association. Cutaneous signs are often mild with, in some cases, an absence of freckling (186). The pathogenesis is different with a postreplication repair defect and normal excision repair. Phototesting with narrow or broadband sources tends to be within normal limits. Management is similar to that of the classic form and essentially preventative with surveillance.

Cockayne syndrome

Both sexes are affected equally by this rare autosomal recessive disease which is characterized by photosensitivity, short stature, mental deficiency, and a range of central nervous system and ocular features.[6,7] Usually in the first year of life, the affected child appears normal. Facial erythema following sunlight exposure, if repetitive, will result in a mottled pigmentation and atrophy. Other skin sites are usually normal. Progressive loss of subcutaneous fat gives the face a cachetic appearance. The limbs tend to be long, hands and ears are disproportionately large, and patients may have a beak nose and a bird-like appearance (187).

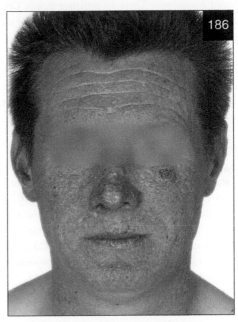

186: Late-onset XP variant in an adult showing minimal XP changes. Note the keratoacanthoma on left upper cheek.
187: Typical dysmorphic features of Cockayne syndrome. (*Reproduced courtesy of St Thomas' Hospital, London.*)

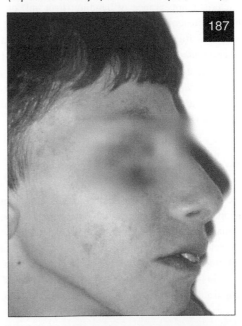

Cataracts, retinal degeneration, and optic atrophy can all result in a progressive loss of vision. Demyelination associated with calcification produces a range of peripheral and central nervous system problems including sensorineural deafness. Rarely associated with survival beyond the second decade, death usually occurs as the result of infection. Some mildly affected patients can live a near normal lifespan. Diagnosis is again made by study of cultured fibroblasts. There is evidence that in Cockayne syndrome patient fibroblasts are hypersensitive to UV killing and also have a specific defect in transcription-coupled repair.

The diagnosis can be made prenatally by molecular genetic testing of a chorionic villus sample. The diagnosis can be difficult with progeria syndromes causing problems. Management is with photoprotection by standard means.

Trichothiodystrophy (TDD)

TDD represents a spectrum of syndromes some of which, but not all, are associated with photosensitivity. All do have specific defects in nucleotide excision repair (NER).[6] All are rare, occur in both sexes, and are inherited as autosomal recessive. The chronic ichthyotic and photosensitivity variant (brittle hair, intellectual impairment, decreased fertility, and short stature – BIDS) can be accompanied by ichthyosis (IBIDS) and increased susceptibility to sunlight (PIBIDS).

In the photosensitive type, there is an excision repair defect with a complementation group identical to that seen in XP (group D). It is curious that no increased susceptibility to skin cancer is seen. The hair, which tends to break easily, has a characteristic appearance of banding (tiger tail) on polarized light microscopy (188).[8] Biochemical assessment of the hair reveals sulfur deficiency when compared with normal hair. In cell mutation studies, fibroblasts reveal XPD. It is of interest that mutations of this specific gene can result in XP, TDD, and the combination of XPD and CS. How this defect produces the characteristics of each condition is unknown. Management is by careful photoprotection.

Defects of DNA helicases

The RecQ family of DNA helicases, which are highly conserved and important for the unwinding of DNA into separate chromatids, have a major role in DNA repair/recombination pathways. A range of defects in this family of enzymes give rise to a number of syndromes, i.e. Rothmund Thomson (RT), Bloom (BS), and progeria (Werner) syndromes (WS). The first two (RT, BS) are recognized to have a significant photosensitivity element.[3]

Rothmund Thomson syndrome (RTS) (poikiloderma congenitale)

This condition, which is rare, occurs in both sexes. As with the other photodermatoses, it has an autosomal recessive inheritance pattern.

It is not a diagnosis that can be made clinically at birth, for the earliest skin abnormalities, which initially can be subtle, present late in the first year or in a few patients over the next two to three years. When fully evident, the features are striking in their morphology and distribution. Early forms may only show an erythema which can be transient. Later the clinically diagnostic finding of marked telangiectasia, atrophy, depigmentation, and patches of pigmentation (poikiloderma), primarily of sunlight-exposed sites of face, legs, arms, and hands, becomes evident (189, 190). Photosensitivity can be severe with bullous lesions following sunlight exposure. In the second and third decades, minor scale, which may become hyperkeratotic/warty and prominent (191), is evident on photo-exposed skin sites. Within these dysplastic areas, squamous cell carcinomas may develop later in life. The histology of affected poikilodermatous skin is not disease specific. Epidermal atrophy may be accompanied by dermo-epidermal junction edema and vasodilatation. Hyperkeratotic lesions often show bowenoid dyskeratosis. In addition to cutaneous squamous cell carcinomas, a significant number of cases develop osteosarcoma.[9] Currently no biologic or molecular markers exist to predict which patients will develop the osteosarcoma, a tumor which, despite improvements in diagnosis, surgery and chemotherapy, still has a substantial mortality rate. Of a group of 41 patients, 32% have been reported as developing this complication.[10] Other extracutaneous features (short stature and skeletal dysplasia) exist and, in a few, there is susceptibility to juvenile bilateral cataracts.

The investigation of a suspected case requires cell mutation study to determine the presence of a deleterious ReCQL4 helicase mutation. Some patients have shown UVA sensitivity on monochromator or broad-spectrum phototesting.

Management is focused on photoprotection with behavioral, clothing, and broad-spectrum sunscreen use. This should be instigated at an early age. Advice on photoprotection at school, including the use of Dermaguard photoprotective film, is important. It is also worth remembering that the early poikilodermatous changes can in part be reversible by avoidance of sunlight.

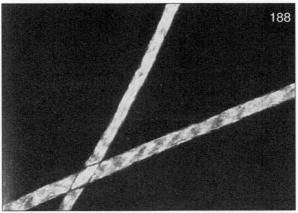

188: Trichothiodystrophy. Typical tiger tail banding seen on hair shafts (under polarized light microscopy).

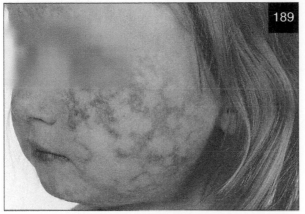

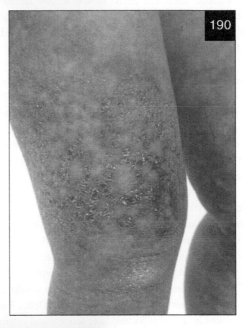

189: Rothmund Thomson syndrome: Young girl with typical poikilodermatous changes on photo-exposed

190: Rothmund Thomson syndrome: Poikiloderma of right thigh and lower leg.

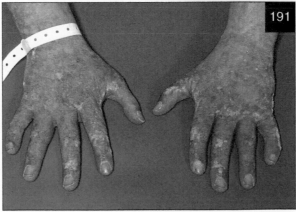

191: Late hyperkeratosis in Rothmund Thomson syndrome.

Bloom syndrome[1]

This extremely rare autosomal recessive disorder, which probably occurs in less than 1:1,000,000 of the UK population, i.e. significantly more uncommon than xeroderma pigmentosum, is characterized by both pre- and postnatal growth retardation that persists with small stature in adult life (**192**). Both sexes are affected equally; carriers are unaffected, and it is known to be commoner in Ashkenazi Jews. Children show a marked recurrent erythema following sunlight exposure, which results in telangiectasia of photo-exposed sites (**193**). In addition, there is evidence that some patients have a degree of immune deficiency. Although females are usually fertile, males are not. The main serious complication of the condition is a marked increase in the incidence of a broad range of malignancies. These include leukemia early in the second decade and breast/GI cancer by the fourth decade. A child who is of small stature with telangiectasia of sunlight-exposed sites should raise the possibility of Bloom syndrome.

It is important that the correct diagnosis be established so that awareness of the malignant potential allows surveillance. Skin biopsy with fibroblast culture will reveal the RecQ helicase enzyme family malfunctions in this condition and increased sister chromatid exchange. How exactly this translates into the salient clinical features of growth retardation, telangiectasia, and the increase in cancer risk is unknown.

Smith–Lemli–Opitz syndrome (SLO)

This rare autosomal recessive, multiple congenital malformation syndrome is caused by a deficiency of cholesterol synthesis at the last step site where 7-dehydrocholesterol is converted into cholesterol by 7-dehydrocholesterol reductase (DHCR7). Deficiency of this enzyme's action results in low levels of cholesterol with high levels of 7-DHC. Initially photosensitivity is not reported; later redness and itching are seen on photosensitive sites. A recent review suggests that more than half of all patients do have a significant photosensitivity which, on phototest investigation, was found to have a UVA dependency (320–400 nm).[11] A large number of different mutations with a range of expressions are detected in cultured fibroblasts. Other clinical features include microcephaly, dysmorphic facies, limb and genital developmental delay, and renal and cardiac malformations. Mild cases with few abnormalities are also reported.

Treatment consists of cholesterol supplementation, which can result in reversal of photosensitivity.

References

1. Woods CG. DNA repair disorders. *Arch Dis Childh* 1998;**78**:178–84.

2. Garfinkel DJ, Bailis AM. Nucleotide excision repair, genome stability, and human disease: new insight from model systems. *J Biomed Biotechnol* 2002;**2**:55–60.

3. Mohaghegh P, Hickson ID. Premature aging in RecQ helicase-deficient human syndromes. *Int J Biochem Cell Biol* 2002;**34**:1496–501.

4. Cleaver JE. Defective repair replication of DNA in xeroderma pigmentosum. *Nature* 1968;**218**:652–6.

5. de Sanctis C, Cacchione A. L'idiozia xerodermica. *Riv Sper Freniatr* 1932;**56**:269.

6. de Boer J, Hoeijmakers JHJ. Nucleotide excision repair and human syndromes. *Carcinogenesis* 2000;**21**:453–60.

7. Olaciregui O, Yoldi ME, Gurtubay IG et al. Clinical and neuropathological study of two brothers with Cockayne Syndrome. *Rev Neurol* 2001;**33**:628–31.

8. Sperling LC, DiGiovanna JJ. "Curly" wood and tiger tails: an explanation for light and dark banding with polarization in trichothiodystrophy. *Arch Dermatol* 2003;**139**:1189–92.

9. Wang LL, Gannavarapu A, Kozinetz CA et al. Association between osteosarcoma and deleterious mutations in the RECQL4 gene in Rothmund–Thomson syndrome. *J Nat Cancer Inst* 2003;**95**:669–74.

10. Wang LL, Levy ML, Lewis RA et al. Clinical manifestations in a cohort of 41 Rothmund-Thomson syndrome patients. *Am J Med Genet* 2001;102:11–17.

11. Anstey A. Photomedicine: lessons from the Smith-Lemli-Opitz syndrome. *J Photochem Photobiol B: Biol* 2001;**62**:123–7.

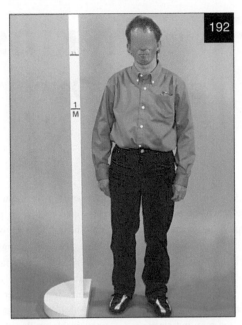

192: Small stature is a feature of Bloom syndrome.

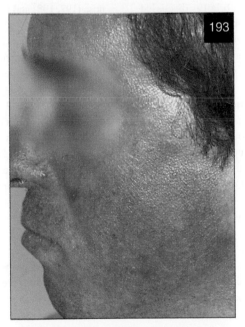

193: Erythema and telangiectasia of photo-exposed sites in Bloom syndrome.

18 The Cutaneous Porphyrias

Robert S Dawe

The porphyrias are a heterogeneous group of conditions caused by inherited or acquired enzyme defects in the porphyrin metabolic pathway (**194**). All the porphyrias except acute intermittent porphyria, and the exceptionally rare aminolevulinic acid dehydratase deficiency porphyria, can affect the skin. In this chapter, the three commonest cutaneous porphyrias in the UK, porphyria cutanea tarda (PCT), erythropoietic protoporphyria (EPP), and variegate porphyria (VP), are discussed. Hereditary coproporphyria and the rare, but severe, congenital erythropoietic porphyria (CEP) and hepato-erythropoietic porphyria are mentioned and briefly discussed. Pseudoporphyria, skin changes similar to those of porphyria cutanea tarda without any biochemical evidence of a porphyria, will be included as it is the most frequent differential diagnosis to be considered when assessing someone with possible PCT.

The porphyrias are classified in various ways: often as "hepatic" or "erythropoietic" based upon where, in which organ, the enzyme defect primarily occurs, or "acute" or "cutaneous" or "mixed" depending upon whether or not acute manifestations of nerve involvement are a feature or not. In this chapter they are classified on the basis of their predominant skin features, that is as:
- porphyrias that typically present with acute phototoxic symptoms (primarily EPP)
- those in which blisters and skin fragility are typical (mainly PCT and VP), and
- the rare, usually congenital, severely scarring (often mutilating) cutaneous porphyrias (particularly CEP).

Acute phototoxic symptoms

Erythropoietic protoporphyria (EPP)

This is the porphyria most frequently investigated in the Dundee Photobiology Unit, although the population prevalence is lower than that for PCT. Its clinical features are very different from those of PCT. It is caused by inherited (autosomal dominant or autosomal recessive) defects in the ferrochelatase gene. The main feature is pain, often described as burning or prickly, in skin exposed to sunlight. As little as a few minutes of intense sunlight is often sufficient to cause symptoms, which occur immediately. Typically the pain is severe and those affected withdraw from further exposure if possible and may try to gain relief from cold water (**195**). Only if further exposure is unavoidable will redness and swelling develop (**196**), and repeated such exposures can lead to typical scarring on dorsal nose (**197, 198**) and thickening of dorsal hand skin.

EPP usually presents in childhood, when the first manifestation may be of a baby crying outdoors or when exposed to sunlight through window-glass. The frequent absence of any physical signs may lead to delay in these symptoms being taken seriously by medical staff, and to delay in diagnosis. Occasionally EPP does not present in childhood and first becomes apparent in adult life, even when the genetic abnormality must have been present since birth. An acquired disorder of ferrochelatase activity, sideroblastic anemia, also needs to be considered if the first symptoms are delayed until adulthood.

The effects of EPP are usually manifest only in the skin. However, as might be expected in a disorder affecting the final step in the heme biosynthetic pathway (**194**), anemia (normochromic, normocytic) may be found. Also, gallstone disease is more frequent than in people without EPP. Hepatocellular liver failure occurs in at most 5% of EPP patients. This seems to be primarily a complication of autosomal recessive EPP.

Treatment consists of advice on measures to minimize sunlight exposure, taking into account that it is the visible wavelengths that cause the skin symptoms. Various free radical scavengers can be used. Traditionally beta-carotene is often prescribed, although a controlled trial showed no clear benefit.

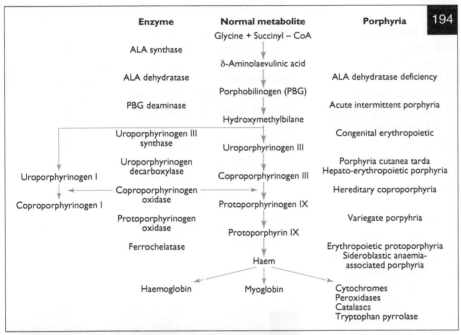

Enzyme	Normal metabolite	Porphyria	194
	Glycine + Succinyl – CoA		
ALA synthase			
ALA dehydratase	δ-Aminolaevulinic acid	ALA dehydratase deficiency	
PBG deaminase	Porphobilinogen (PBG)	Acute intermittent porphyria	
	Hydroxymethylbilane		
Uroporphyrinogen III synthase		Congenital erythropoietic	
Uroporphyrinogen decarboxylase	Uroporphyrinogen III	Porphyria cutanea tarda Hepato-erythropoietic porphyria	
Coproporphyrinogen oxidase	Coproporphyrinogen III	Hereditary coproporphyria	
Protoporphyrinogen oxidase	Protoporphyrinogen IX	Variegate porpyhria	
Ferrochelatase	Protoporphyrin IX	Erythropoietic protoporphyria Sideroblastic anaemia-associated porphyria	
	Haem		

Uroporphyrinogen I

Coproporphyrinogen I

Haemoglobin   Myoglobin   Cytochromes
Peroxidases
Catalascs
Tryptophan pyrrolase

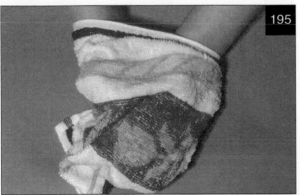

194: The porphyrin-heme biosynthetic pathway.

195: The pain of sites exposed to sunlight in EPP is often described as "stinging" or "burning". Applying a towel soaked in cold water or holding exposed sites under a running cold tap are typical responses to EPP pain (which is similar to the pain associated with topical ALA-photodynamic therapy [see Chapter 16]).

196: Slight redness and swelling of sunlight exposed sites. Apparently disproportionate symptoms associated with often rather subtle clinical signs are common in EPP. The redness will often start while exposed and tends to peak quickly and resolve quickly (a different time course from that of sunburn erythema).

197: Episode of crusting on nose and swelling and redness of upper lip and philtrum in EPP.

198: Repeated such episodes can result in this pattern of scarring.

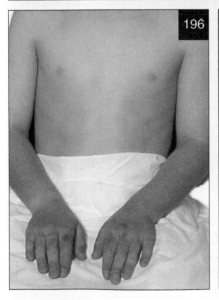

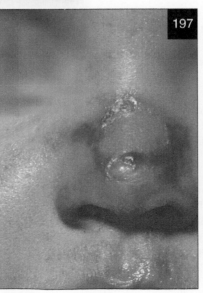

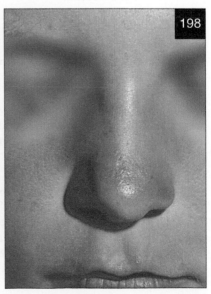

Sideroblastic anemia-associated porphyrias

Reports of porphyria associated with sideroblastic anemia and myelodysplasia describe two main patterns of porphyria, which are sometimes combined. One is associated with acquired reduced ferrochelatase activity, and results in the same skin symptoms and signs as erythropoietic protoporphyria, and the other is porphyria cutanea tarda secondary to iron overload caused by blood transfusions.

Blisters and skin fragility

Porphyria cutanea tarda (PCT)

This is the commonest of the cutaneous porphyrias in Europe, and probably worldwide. Its estimated prevalence was 1 in 5000 of the population in the former Czechoslovakia. PCT is important not only in its own right, but because sporadic PCT is a marker for liver disease and an increased risk of hepatocellular carcinoma. PCT is caused by a reduction in the activity of uroporphyrinogen decarboxylase, the fifth enzyme in the porphyrin pathway (**194**). The rare PCT types 2 and 3 are due to different inherited patterns of this enzyme deficiency. Most cases of PCT fall into the "sporadic" or "acquired" (type 1) group. In some of these patients there may be a contributory inherited low activity of uroporphyrinogen decarboxylase, but liver disease is necessary to reduce this enzyme level sufficiently for PCT to develop. When chronic hepatitis induces PCT, liver iron overload is usually present, and heterozygosity for a hemochromatosis gene is contributory to the development of PCT in many of those affected. The most frequent causes of PCT in Europe are:

- excessive alcohol intake
- chronic hepatitis C infection
- other chronic viral infections that affect the liver (including HIV)
- autoimmune chronic hepatitis (for example, in SLE), and
- hemochromatosis.

Medications are not as important as triggers as in the acute porphyrias (see below), but estrogens are thought to play a part in inducing PCT in some people and treatment with iron will exacerbate PCT.

Sporadic PCT usually first develops over the age of 40, and is commoner in men than women. The most frequent presentation is with blisters and skin fragility on maximally photo-exposed sites of dorsal hands (**199, 200**). The subepidermal blisters of PCT typically result in milia (**201, 202**). Another frequent feature is hypertrichosis, often first noticeable on temples but not restricted to photo-exposed sites. Pigmentation, particularly of photo-exposed sites, is another common feature, which is occasionally the sole presenting sign. Solar urticaria is uncommon as a presenting feature, although urticarial responses can more often be produced when the patient is being phototested (**203**). Scleroderma-like changes are not commonly seen, but are well described in PCT (**204**). Many people with PCT are not aware of the role of sunlight. This is because:

- it is visible (not ultraviolet) wavelength radiation that causes the skin changes so seasonal variation is not always evident
- it is mainly chronic exposure, and not discrete episodes in sunlight, that is most important.

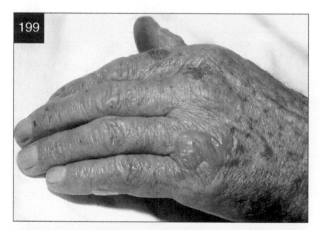

199: Unilocular large intact bulla (reflecting subepidermal cleft) in PCT.

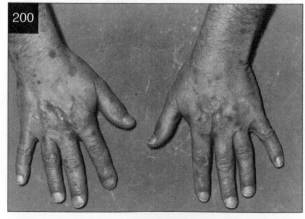

200: Post-inflammatory changes reflecting previous blisters, and erosions, on typical maximally photo-exposed sites of dorsal hands.

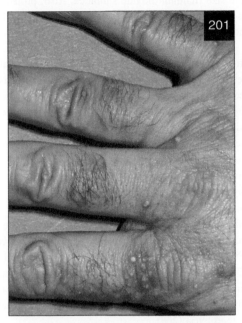

201: Small milia in PCT.

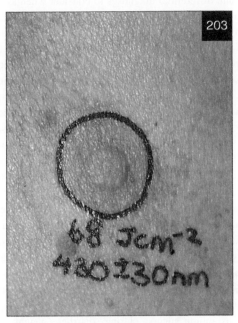

203: Blue light irradiation-induced immediate urticarial response in a patient with PCT. This patient did not have symptomatic solar urticaria.

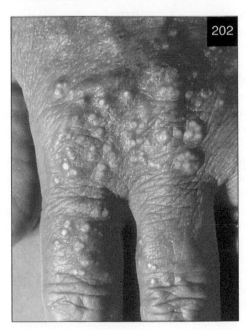

202: More numerous milia in PCT.

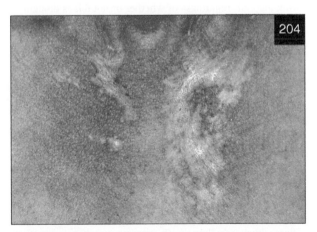

204: Photo-exposed localized morphea as a manifestation of PCT. More severe widespread progressive morphea has occasionally been associated with PCT.

The main differential diagnoses to consider when assessing a patient presenting with typical features are variegate porphyria, hereditary coproporphyria, and drug-induced pseudoporphyria (Chapter 15). A peak around 618 nm to 620 nm on plasma spectrofluorimetry (see Chapter 16) confirms the diagnosis, which can be corroborated by quantification of urine and stool porphyrins (205). Urinary porphyrin concentrations can be used to help monitor the response to therapy. In an unusually young patient (<30 years old) presenting with PCT, the primarily inherited PCT types 2 and 3 should be considered. In the majority the diagnosis is type 1 sporadic PCT and after making this diagnosis, it is necessary to investigate to determine what liver insults have caused it and whether or not there is clear evidence of iron overload. Investigations required for all patients include transaminases, hepatitis B and C serology, ferritin, and alfa-fetoprotein. In areas of high HIV prevalence, HIV serology should always be checked. In low-prevalence areas, the threshold for requesting HIV serology should be low, and it should be checked whether there are other pointers to this diagnosis (such as mouth ulcers, chronic diarrhea, weight loss or behavioral risk factors) or if the PCT presentation is unusual (for example, in a young woman who drinks little alcohol).

Management involves treating the causes of underlying hepatitis when possible. Patients should be advised not to drink alcohol (regardless of whether or not this is thought to be the primary liver insult), and medications containing iron and estrogens must be stopped. When possible, viral hepatitis should be treated, with interferon for hepatitis C or combination antiretroviral chemotherapy for HIV. The likelihood of treatment of hepatitis C being effective is increased if iron overload is addressed first. Iron overload is usually treated by venesection. Iron chelation therapy (with desferrioxamine) is an alternative approach, which is particularly useful when iron overload is associated with anemia (such as in a hemodialysis patient with hepatitis C-induced PCT). Another approach, which can be combined with venesection, is to treat with low-dose hydroxychloroquine or chloroquine.

These drugs are thought to increase porphyrin excretion. Sunlight avoidance measures are important while the effects of these treatments are awaited. Patients need to reduce visible light exposure, by behavioral avoidance, appropriate clothing (for example, dark-colored driving gloves), and using a large-particle size titanium dioxide sunblock. Also, protection of hands from trauma by wearing gloves during manual work and hobby activities (such as gardening) usually helps.

Pseudoporphyria and porphyria of renal failure

These are, by definition, not true porphyrias, that is diseases caused by reduced activity of one or more enzymes in the porphyrin-heme biosynthetic pathway. However, they are included here because they are conditions that clinically mimic PCT (and the skin manifestations of variegate porphyria) (206). Pseudoporphyria is usually caused by a drug, with naproxen the commonest single drug to cause pseudoporphyria investigated in the Dundee Photobiology Unit (207). Naproxen pseudoporphyria can persist for over a year after the drug is stopped. A PCT-like presentation in hemodialyzed renal failure patients is more complicated: it can be true PCT (perhaps triggered by iatrogenically acquired hepatitis C infection in the past) or a condition of abnormal porphyrin biochemistry caused by impaired elimination (but without an enzyme defect) or it can be drug-induced pseudoporphyria (208).

Variegate porphyria (VP)

The skin manifestations of VP (209) can be identical to those of PCT. It is important to recognize because neurovisceral attacks, as in acute intermittent porphyria, may occur. The diagnosis of PCT is strongly suggested if the porphyrin plasma scan peak is at 626 nm, but (because of the implications of the diagnosis for patient and family) the diagnosis should be confirmed with quantitative urine and stool porphyrin biochemistry. The porphyrin plasma scan is a useful screening test for family members of a VP patient, although false negatives are more likely under age 14 years. As with the other acute porphyrias (acute intermittent porphyria and hereditary coproporphyria being the others most frequently encountered in the UK) many drugs can trigger acute attacks. The list of porphyrinogenic drugs in the British National Formulary is helpful.

Hereditary coproporphyria

This is very uncommon but the skin features are reported to be similar to those of PCT. It is important because acute neurovisceral attacks can occur, and the plasma scan peak can be identical to that of PCT, so the diagnosis can only be established (or excluded) by quantification of fecal porphyrins.

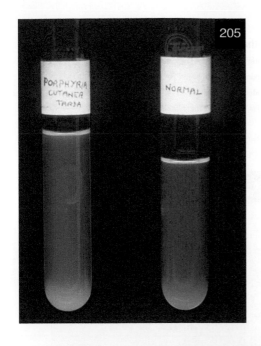

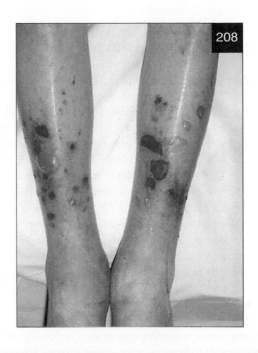

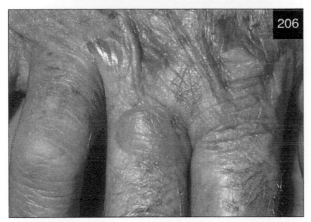

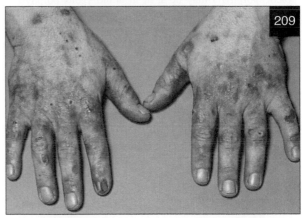

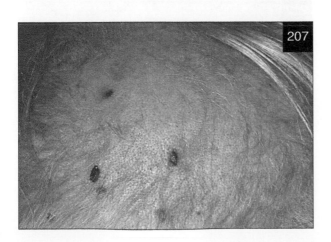

205: Although plasma spectrofluorimetry is the screening test of choice if readily accessible (because it not only helps confirm PCT when this is suspected but also differentiates PCT from variegate porphyria), simply examining urine under a Wood's lamp is a very simple screening test that can be done in any clinic.

206: This patient had naproxen-induced pseudoporphyria: these clinical findings are identical to those of PCT or variegate porphyria. A normal porphyrin plasma scan, and knowledge that he had been on naproxen for 6 months, made the diagnosis.

207: Skin fragility, resulting in these photo-exposed site erosions on scalp, persistent 1 year after naproxen was stopped.

208: Pseudoporphyria from frusemide treatment in a renal failure patient.

209: Erosions, blisters, and postinflammatory changes on dorsal hands. (The right index finger nail dystrophy is probably unrelated.)

Severe scarring porphyrias

Congenital erythropoietic porphyria (Günther's porphyria) is a very rare autosomal recessive porphyria. Late-onset, mild expression cases have been reported but it usually presents in infancy. Pink or dark brown staining of nappies may be noted from a very high urinary uroporphyrin I concentration. Affected infants may, like those with erythropoietic protoporphyria (EPP), cry if exposed to sunlight or phototherapy for hyperbilirubinemia. The photosensitivity is, however, usually much more severe than in EPP and episodes of redness and swelling usually occur, resulting in blistering and then scarring causing mutilation of ears, nose and fingers. Scarring alopecia typically develops on the scalp (**210**), hypertrichosis may be severe, and teeth will be brown and fluoresce under Wood's lamp. A hemolytic anemia resulting in splenomegaly is often a feature of the condition.

Similarly severe, mutilating skin changes to those of erythropoietic porphyria may be seen in homozygous porphyrias, such as homozygous variegate porphyria (**210, 211, 212**) and homozygous PCT (hepatoerythropoietic porphyria).

Further Reading

1. Murphy, G.M., The cutaneous porphyrias: a review. The British Photodermatology Group. *Br J Dermatol*, 1999. **140**(4): p. 573-81.
2. Badminton, M.N. and G.H. Elder, Management of acute and cutaneous porphyrias. *Int J Clin Pract*, 2002. **56**(4): p. 272-8.

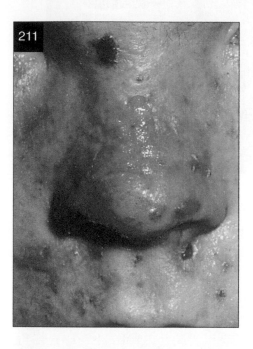

211: Homozygote variegate porphyria: note the scarring as well as ongoing erosions and ulceration.

212: Homozygous variegate porphyria: the severity of these changes (in a child in a temperate country) argues against PCT or VP.

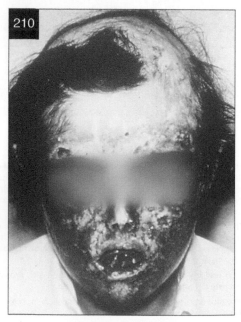

210: Adult with erythropoietic porphyria.

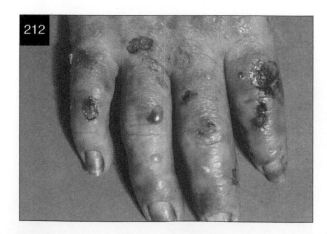

19
Ultraviolet Phototherapy and Photochemotherapy of Skin Disease
David Bilsland and Robert S Dawe

Ultraviolet radiation therapy is used for a wide variety of skin diseases. Currently, the two main treatment approaches *(Table 19.1)* are:

- phototherapy with ultraviolet B (UVB) (**213**), either narrowband (311 nm–313 nm) UVB phototherapy or lamps emitting a broader spectrum of UVB and ultraviolet A (broadband UVB, BB-UVB)
- psoralen photochemotherapy using UVA after oral or topical administration of a photosensitizing psoralen (psoralen-UVA, PUVA).

This chapter describes the most frequent indications for UVB and PUVA, and the factors that need to be taken into account when you are deciding to prescribe one of these treatments. We then discuss how these treatments are administered, followed by comment on adverse effects (common and infrequent but serious). Brief mention is made of other forms of phototherapy that are not presently established treatments in most UK centers, particularly ultraviolet A1 (UVA1).

The most frequent indications for UVB in the UK are psoriasis, atopic dermatitis, and polymorphic light eruption (for which phototherapy is given as prophylaxis, rather than to suppress an established eruption). The main indications for PUVA are similar. For the diseases most commonly treated, controlled studies form the evidence base, but for treatment of rarer conditions the evidence for use of UVB or PUVA comes from case series rather than controlled studies *(Table 19.2)*.

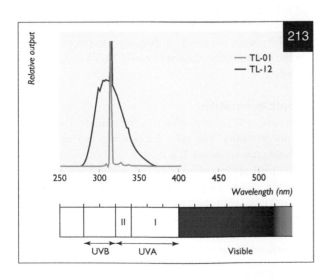

213: Emission spectra of typical broadband UVB (Philips TL-12) and narrowband UVB (Philips TL-01) lamps.

Table 19.1: Definitions

- Phototherapy: the therapeutic use of non-ionizing electromagnetic radiation.
- UVB: 290–320 nm
- UV: 320–400 nm
- UVA2: 320–340 nm 2
- UVA1: 340–400 nm 1
- Photochemotherapy: the therapeutic use of non-ionizing radiation in combination with a photosensitizing drug.

Table 19.2: Indications for UVB and PUVA

Condition	Comment
Established major indications	
Psoriasis	Consider PUVA if UVB disappointing (for example, short remission)
Atopic dermatitis	PUVA very rarely justified in childhood (but consider before systemic immunosuppression)
Polymorphic light eruption	PUVA is more effective than broadband UVB, so consider if narrowband UVB unavailable
Vitiligo	UVB (narrowband) probably as effective as PUVA
Mycosis fungoides	UVB for patch stage; PUVA for plaque stage
Other indications (less frequently treated, less evidence of effectiveness)	
Dermatitis other than atopic dermatitis	Very limited study evidence: UVB to be preferred, except for palm and sole dermatoses for which PUVA may be better
Chronic urticarias	Limited study evidence
Acne vulgaris	Broadband UVB at erythemogenic doses (mainly of historic interest now that more effective therapies are available)
Pityriasis rosea	UVB effective but rarely required
Pityriasis lichenoides chronica	UVB treatment of choice
Generalized itch	Good evidence for efficacy of UVB particularly in itch of kidney failure, but can be useful even for "idiopathic pruritus"
Lichen planus	No comparative studies, but narrowband UVB often effective for widespread disease; PUVA for severe palmar involvement
Granuloma annulare	Both UVB and PUVA may clear this
Necrobiosis lipoidica	PUVA possibly effective (ulcer healing, and perhaps changing texture towards normal, as well as camouflaging)
Pityriasis rubra pilaris	PUVA sometimes useful; almost invariably exacerbated by UVB

Indications for UVB or PUVA

Psoriasis

Psoriasis (**214, 215**) is the most common indication for UVB and for PUVA. PUVA is more effective than broadband UVB, but not much different in efficacy compared to narrowband UVB. In general, PUVA is used only when UVB, administered appropriately, fails to adequately clear psoriasis or when the duration of remission is short. In view of the cumulative exposure-related skin cancer risks known to be associated with PUVA, UVB is preferred, particularly for younger patients. Neither therapy is curative, and remissions of on average 6 months can be expected *(Table 19.3)*.

When is UVB indicated?

- For patients who have extensive disease on limbs and body which makes practical use of topical therapy difficult.
- If topical therapy has not worked.

When should PUVA be used instead of UVB?

- If UVB is ineffective.
- If the duration of remission following three consecutive UVB courses is consistently short (for example, <2 months).
- For palmoplantar pustular psoriasis, PUVA appears more effective.

Atopic dermatitis

UVB and PUVA are effective treatments for atopic eczema/dermatitis. The rules for psoriasis can broadly be applied to this condition. It is used:

- for particularly extensive truncal and limb eczema
- when standard topical therapies are not controlling activity or only resulting in short-term remissions
- as steroid-sparing therapy when potent or very potent topical steroids are otherwise required continuously to maintain disease control.

As for psoriasis PUVA should be reserved for older patients and those who are not helped by UVB. In general, treatment courses often have to be more gentle, with lower increments and more prolonged in comparison to those used for psoriasis *(Table 19.4)*.

Topical therapy with corticosteroids should be continued, although the need for this will reduce as the disease is brought under control with phototherapy. If your phototherapy

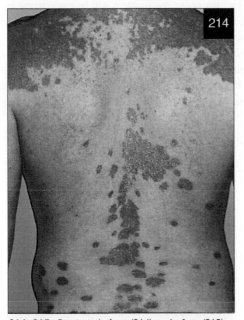

214, 215: Psoriasis before (214) and after (215) a course of narrowband UVB.

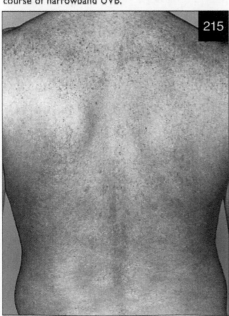

department is not air-conditioned, then heat particularly in the summer months may be a reason for apparent treatment failure, because sweating can be a factor in aggravating the eczema.

Polymorphic light eruption

Mild polymorphic light eruption (PLE) (see Chapter 5) is usually managed with advice on behavioral, clothing, and topical sunscreen photoprotection measures. However, when it is more severe and impairing life quality, prophylactic PUVA or UVB phototherapy administered in spring is beneficial. Narrowband UVB is as effective as PUVA, and generally preferable for its convenience and greater safety. However, PUVA is more effective than broadband UVB. Patients need to know before starting treatment that it is common for PLE to be provoked during the course. This can usually be managed by adjusting the doses used, treating only sites requiring therapy (for example, treating patients wearing shorts and a T-shirt, the same ones each treatment), and if necessary applying a potent topical corticosteroid immediately after each treatment. If PLE is very readily provoked by UVB, then PUVA may be better, and vice versa. Reasons for failure are given in *Table 19.5.*

Table 19.3: Phototherapy for psoriasis

- Narrowband UVB is more effective than broadband UVB for psoriasis.
- Narrowband UVB and PUVA are of similar efficacy for psoriasis.
- For convenience and safety reasons narrowband UVB is the first choice phototherapy for psoriasis.

Table 19.4: Phototherapy for atopic dermatitis

- Phototherapy for atopic dermatitis requires a "gentler" regimen than for psoriasis.
- It is important that flares of atopic dermatitis are treated as usual during a phototherapy course.
- Although one indication for phototherapy for atopic dermatitis is to reduce topical steroid requirements, it is important that these are not withdrawn too early.
- Improvement of atopic dermatitis with phototherapy is often not apparent until 15–20 treatments have been given.

Table 19.5: Common reasons for "failure" of prophylactic phototherapy for PLE

- Given at suboptimal time of year (too early or too late).
- Attempts to treat normally covered sites that do not require treatment.
- Failure to manage induced PLE during a treatment course (with dose adjustments, topical corticosteroids immediately after treatments if necessary).

Cutaneous T cell lymphoma (mycosis fungoides)

The effect of PUVA on the long-term prognosis of cutaneous T cell lymphoma (CTCL) is unknown. The finding of "solar signature" *p53* mutations in tumor stage CTCL raises possible concerns about use of phototherapy and photochemotherapy, although there is no evidence to suggest that treatment with either adversely affects the natural history. If simple treatment approaches with topical steroids have been unhelpful, PUVA is an effective treatment for symptomatic (pruritic) early stage I and Ia patch and plaque disease *(Table 19.6)*. The effect appears to be localized to exposed sites, and "sanctuary site" disease does not clear (**216, 217**). It is also useful, sometimes in combination with other therapies such as retinoids or interferon, in the palliation of later stage disease. Narrowband UVB is effective for patch stage disease but once lesions are palpably thickened PUVA is more likely to be effective.

Table 19.6: Phototherapy for mycosis fungoides

- No treatments for mycosis fungoides are known to alter prognosis.
- The simplest safest treatment that controls symptoms should be chosen.

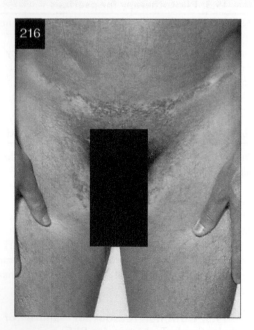

Vitiligo

Narrowband UVB and PUVA can both induce repigmentation. Up to 70% of patients with vitiligo benefit if they are treated continuously for a year or more. Those with trichrome pattern vitiligo, that is those with areas of reduced pigment as well as areas of normal skin and of complete pigment loss, tend to respond better. Acral sites respond poorly. Patients repigment in a perifollicular fashion initially (**218**). In patients with skin phototypes II–V, there is a danger that, if complete repigmentation does not occur, the problem will be made worse by exaggeration of contrast between vitiligo and surrounding skin, and there could be scattered macules of follicular pigment if partial repigmentation occurs. However, if the patient is well motivated, has a good understanding of their condition and what to expect from this treatment, and has a pattern of vitiligo that is likely to respond, then UVB or PUVA can greatly

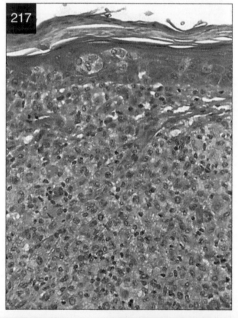

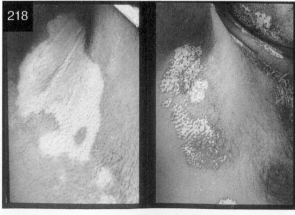

216: Sanctuary site mycosis fungoides developing in sites covered by genital protection worn during PUVA by this patient whose mycosis fungoides elsewhere cleared well.

217: Histopathology of biopsy taken from sanctuary site skin shown in 19.3.

218: Vitiligo responding to narrowband UVB phototherapy. Note the follicular pigmentation and the accentuation of brown pigment around the lesion's periphery – patients must be warned this often occurs with PUVA (probably less often with NB-UVB) and can make affected skin areas more noticeable.

improve quality of life. Some of those in whom successful repigmentation is achieved keep their pigmentation after an initial prolonged course of treatment, but others lose it again and require repeated courses *(Table 19.7)*.

It should be remembered that a course of PUVA for vitiligo may easily give a patient a high cumulative dose with 150–200 treatments given twice weekly over 1–2 years. A frank discussion with the patient of the risks of therapy – the risk of more pronounced lesional adverse effects with "burning" and blistering, and the possibility of an increased skin cancer risk compared to unaffected skin – is a must before embarking on prolonged courses of phototherapy for vitiligo.

Contraindications to UVB or PUVA

There are a few absolute contraindications, particularly in those who:

- are medically unfit – for example, those with severe cardiovascular or respiratory disease that prevents standing in the treatment cubicle, or that could be destabilized should an unexpected sunburn-like erythema occur
- have lupus erythematosus
- have genophotodermatoses, for example xeroderma pigmentosum (see Chapter 17)
- are pregnant (a contraindication to systemic PUVA, but not to UVB).

Relative contraindications include:

- a personal history of skin cancer
- those with atypical nevus syndrome
- a family history of skin cancer (melanoma or non-melanoma skin cancers at an unusually young age)
- previous exposure to radiotherapy
- medications that may interact with psoralens (for PUVA), or that may be photo-active in UVB range (for UVB) (these are usually not a problem as long as pretreatment minimal phototoxic dose (for PUVA) or minimal erythemal dose (for UVB) testing is performed
- young age, because of long-term risks – PUVA should usually be avoided in children
- those with photo-induced epilepsy or poorly controlled epilepsy – well-controlled epilepsy, not known to be triggered by fluorescent lamp exposure, is not a contraindication, but the nurse phototherapist needs to be in line of eye and verbal contact with the cubicle during treatment to ensure patient safety.

Table 19.7: Phototherapy for vitiligo

- Narrowband UVB and PUVA can both be effective for vitiligo.
- Prolonged courses are required.
- Therefore, patients must be well motivated, knowledgeable about the likelihood of success or failure, and fully aware of potential adverse effects.

How are phototherapy and photochemotherapy administered?

Before starting treatment with UVB or PUVA
Patient assessment
The patient is referred from the dermatology outpatient clinic to the phototherapy unit with a completed referral and consent form. A risk factor profile including previous phototherapy or PUVA treatments, sun exposure history, occupation, personal and family history of skin cancer, and medication taken during the previous 6 months is included in the information on this form. Examination establishes disease extent, and any evidence of photodamage, nevi, any skin cancers or precancerous lesions (such as solar keratoses), and vitiligo is recorded.

Patient education
An information sheet explains the treatment protocol, advises use of appropriate emollients (that is, emollients without sun barrier properties, and also without fragrances or other possibly photo-active ingredients), and explains both acute and chronic adverse effects of treatment. The treatment cabinet is demonstrated, and advice given on the need for consistency of hairstyle and dress during the course of phototherapy to avoid unexpected erythema reactions. Patients are asked to sign a consent form before beginning treatment.

Dosimetry
For hospital-based practice, if there is a local medical physics department, then it is important that UVB and UVA cubicle outputs are regularly checked with an appropriately calibrated meter, used according to standardized methods, and that checks are made whenever the cubicle output might have changed significantly – for example, if more than one or two lamps need to be changed. Only if outputs are measured accurately is it possible to be sure that doses are being administered as prescribed. It has been our experience that in-built cabinet dosimeters can be unreliable, although for office-based practice they may have to be relied upon if there is not ready access to external calibration checks.

According to local protocols we regularly check the irradiance of all phototherapy equipment, and whenever tubes are changed, and with the use of the simple formula below we amend a table of doses and corresponding exposure times accordingly (see Chapter 3).

irradiance (mW/cm²) x time (seconds) = dose (mJ/cm²)

Documentation

The dose given, adverse effects, and response to treatment are recorded at each visit. The cumulative dose, numbers of exposures, adverse effects, and efficacy of treatment are typed into the database and a summary sheet is placed at the front of the phototherapy notes. When the patient finishes a course of phototherapy (or PUVA) a copy of this summary sheet is put in the patient's main hospital notes.

UVB phototherapy regimen

Treatment regimen

The optimum treatment regimen for each UVB-responsive condition has yet to be defined. However, recent and ongoing research should ensure that, in the future, the use of UVB phototherapy is based even more firmly on evidence, rather than anecdote and tradition.

It is useful to consider the various variables that alter treatment efficacy and safety, in conjunction with the ideals we are aiming for when prescribing UVB.

Variables in UVB phototherapy

These include:
- ultraviolet source - the properties of the lamps used, especially the spectrum of wavelengths emitted
- starting dose
- treatment frequency
- dose increments.

Our aim is to adjust the above variables to achieve:
- effective clearance of the condition, with prolonged remission
- minimization of side effects (both acute and chronic)
- low cumulative number of exposures to clearance (and over each patient's lifetime)
- low cumulative dose
- short exposure times
- low cost.

Other factors influencing the treatment regimen include:
- condition treated, and
- patient characteristics, for example skin phototype.

Over the past decade, most progress has been made in the treatment of psoriasis, the condition for which we have most evidence about how to use UVB phototherapy. We know that:
- the narrowband UVB lamp is more effective than broadband UVB. While narrowband UVB in common with all UVB sources will predictably produce erythema, it appears to be the case that suberythemogenic doses will clear psoriasis (see the next two points). On the basis of evidence from animal studies and knowledge of how the treatment is currently used, it is likely (but not certain) to prove safer regarding long-term non-melanoma skin cancer risk
- on safety grounds, and for patient convenience (avoiding unnecessary visits to the department), we base our starting dose on a percentage of each individual's minimal erythema dose (MED)
- a recent study comparing a low and a high incremental dosage regimen favored the low incremental dosage regimen (which is shown below)
- for the majority of patients (of Fitzpatrick skin phototypes I–III of a Northern European population) a three-times weekly treatment is to be preferred to a five-times weekly treatment.

A current standard treatment regimen is shown in *Table 19.8*. Expected average (median) number of exposures for effective treatment is shown in *Table 19.9*.

Table 19.8: Standard UVB phototherapy regimen

Dose	Amount
Initial	50% or 70% of MED*
Subsequent doses (thrice weekly)	psoriasis (in increments of 20%** of previous dose) atopic eczema (in increments of 20%** of previous dose) desensitization (in increments of 20%** of previous dose)

*The optimal percentage of MED starting dose has not been determined).
** Reducing to 10%, depending on erythema response: it is important to ask about reactions to previous treatment, and make a skin examination. This can be done usually by an experienced phototherapy nurse in a well-lit room, at each visit.

Minimal erythema dose (MED) determination

Ideally, an attempt should be made to individualize the starting dose by basing it on MED assessment. In the UK, the MED is defined as the dose of radiation that produces minimal erythema at 24 hours post irradiation. Elsewhere, a different definition (the dose that causes well-defined erythema) is used. There is a poor correlation between the MED and skin type. Determining the MED allows a safe, but not too low, UV starting dose to be administered to each patient. Although the most frequent acute adverse effect that can be avoided by basing starting dose on the MED is erythema, occasionally

the MED testing reveals unexpected severe photosensitivity, such as solar urticaria (219) or chronic actinic dermatitis. Such testing may also show the papular response typical of polymorphic light eruption. (220).

It may be impractical in some units to perform MEDs and an empiric starting dose may be used. This should be carefully chosen based on knowledge of the local skin type population and should always be well below the likely erythemal threshold for the majority of patients.

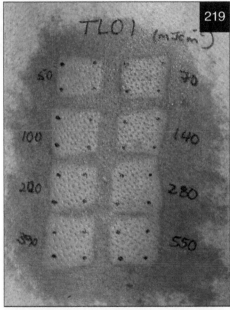

219: Solar urticaria unexpectedly revealed in a night-worker about to start narrowband UVB for atopic dermatitis.

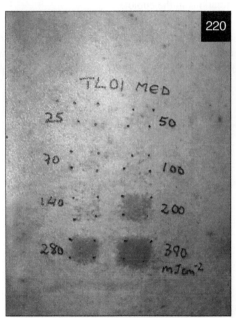

220: This patient was about to start prophylactic treatment for polymorphic light eruption, but this papular response (most marked at 140 mJ/cm²) is also seen from time to time on MED-testing patients about to start treatment for other conditions, such as psoriasis. A response like this does not preclude effective and safe NB-UVB phototherapy but indicates that caution may be required with dose increments (particularly in the psoriasis patient who is a positive Köbner reactor).

Table 19.9: **Expected average (median) number of exposures for effective treatment**

Condition	Median number of exposures
Psoriasis	20–25
Atopic eczema	30–35
Polymorphic light eruption	15
Chronic urticaria	35
Generalized pruritus	25

Method

If a separate irradiation source (**221**) is used to determine the MED, it must contain the same type of lamps as those in the UVB cabinet, and dosimetry must be accurate. In some centers the treatment cabinet itself is used (**222**), although this has disadvantages:

- treatments cannot be given while MED assessment irradiations are performed
- it is time-consuming to cover patients up adequately to safely perform MED irradiations in the cubicle
- some patients (for example, young children and claustrophobic people) may be unable to cope with MED irradiations in the cubicle.

MED is usually determined on back, forearm or buttock skin (preferred site varies between units). In Dundee, a template of eight 1 x 1 cm squares is affixed to the back of the patient and each square is exposed to a different dose of radiation. The remainder of the patient must be covered during these exposures. The selection of exposure doses is based on the skin type of the individual. For example, for narrowband UVB, doses of 25, 50, 70, 100, 140, 200, 280, 390 mJ/cm^2 (Dundee doses, external meter calibration) are used for skin phototype I and II patients, but the first two doses are omitted and doses of 550 and 770 mJ/cm^2 added for higher phototype patients. The erythemal response to these exposures is evaluated at 24 hours. Note the geometric series of doses chosen: there are theoretic reasons, based on the UVB-erythema dose-response curve, to use such a series and not a straight arithmetic series. In practice, the main problem with a simple arithmetic series is that with most such series (for example, 70, 80, 90, 100, 110, 120 mJ/cm^2) the maximum dose will be below the MED for a significant minority of patients, who will be under-treated as a result.

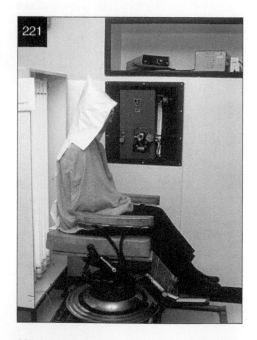

221: Using a bank of narrow-band UVB lamps separate from the cubicles used for treatment makes MED testing more convenient for patients and staff and, in a sufficiently staffed unit, allows MED testing to be conducted while phototherapy for other patients is ongoing. It does require careful dosimetry to ensure that doses administered using the separate bank of lamps correspond to those that will be administered in the treatment cubicle.

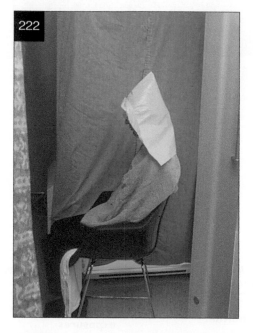

222: MED testing using the door of a treatment cubicle where a separate bank of the appropriate tubes was not available.

Why assess MED?

The starting dose is not routinely based on MED determination, which does require accurate dosimetry and well-trained staff, in all centers. However, when practicable, the starting dose should be MED based as assessing the MED allows us to:

- give an individualized, appropriate dose to each patient
- maximize therapy and therefore reduce number of exposures required to clear
- allow for photo-active medication
- allow for tanning or extensive vitiligo (MED being assessed on a patch of vitiligo)
- identify unsuspected photodermatoses, for example lupus erythematosus, chronic actinic dermatitis syndrome or solar urticaria.

Potential pitfalls in assessing the MED

We use the following points to guide treatment.

- Oral or topical steroid therapy will suppress the erythema response to radiation.
- The mid-back is generally the favored site because the forearm registers a higher MED.
- If a patient is tanned, one must take into account any non-pigmented sites (for example, buttocks or patches of vitiligo). The starting dose of UVB for vitiligo should whenever possible be based on determining the MED on a depigmented patch.

PUVA photochemotherapy regimen

Choice of psoralen and its route of administration

The psoralen most widely used is 8-methoxypsoralen (8-MOP), administered by mouth. If the microcrystalline tablet formulation is used, UVA treatment is usually given 2 hours after the tablets (0.6 mg/kg or a dose based on a surface area nomogram) are taken. Nausea is a frequent side effect of 8-MOP: this is usually not a problem if the tablets are taken with food, but some patients need to be changed to 5-methoxypsoralen (5-MOP) tablets which rarely, if ever, cause this adverse effect. It is because it is not certain that 5-MOP PUVA is as effective as 8-MOP PUVA (and 5-MOP is more expensive) that 8-MOP is generally the standard first-line psoralen.

The psoralen can also be administered topically, by application as a bath-water solution for whole-body treatment or as soaks, paint or cream for localized treatment (for example, for hands and feet). In the UK, 8-MOP is the psoralen currently most widely used for bath PUVA, although in some areas trimethylpsoralen (TMP) is favored. Bath PUVA is more time-consuming for patients and staff than oral PUVA, but may be preferred when the patient is on medications, such as warfarin, which might interact with an oral psoralen or if the eye protection necessary for oral PUVA will be particularly problematic. Also, when psoralens are applied topically they reach a higher skin concentration, and shorter UVA exposures are needed for the same effect: this is particularly true for TMP, and is an advantage if short treatment times are important (for example, for very frail or claustrophobic patients), but can be a disadvantage in that the risk of phototoxic erythema reactions after natural sunlight UVA exposure is greater.

Starting dose – minimal phototoxic dose (MPD) determination

The starting dose should ideally be based on each individual's minimal phototoxic dose. The reasons for doing this are similar to those described for performing MED testing before UVB phototherapy. Additionally, for oral PUVA, MPD assessment ensures that the psoralen dose given does cause a phototoxic reaction. If it does not then MPD testing should be repeated after an increased psoralen dose or a switch to topical PUVA made. Although not ideal, oral PUVA is sometimes started at a low UVA dose without prior MPD determination. Bath PUVA should never be started without the MPD being determined first because of the particularly severe photosensitivity that can result, and which cannot be predicted by skin phototype or any other patient characteristics.

Frequency of treatment

Treatment with PUVA is normally twice weekly (based on the time course of PUVA erythema, which peaks later than UVB erythema), although in some countries thrice-weekly treatment is customary. When necessary for patient convenience, once-weekly treatment can also be effective, although it takes longer to see benefit.

Special precautions

Patients treated with PUVA need to be careful to avoid natural UV exposure (including exposure through window-glass and cloud) throughout the course. Following psoralen tablets, eye protection (UVA-absorbing spectacles) is advised for 24 hours, and following bath psoralen application if an inflammatory dermatosis treated is very extensive (and significant systemic absorption possible), to minimize the risk that a psoralen-UVA reaction in eye lenses could lead to cataracts.

Adjuvant therapy (UVB and PUVA)

With an optimal phototherapy or PUVA regimen for psoriasis, there is generally little therapeutic advantage in using topical therapies such as coal tar, salicylic acid, dithranol or calcipotriol. Most patients welcome the break from daily topical treatments when they attend for phototherapy. However, for some patients, and for "stubborn" psoriasis plaques, such adjunctive therapy can be useful. The study evidence particularly supports the use of calcipotriol as an adjunct to PUVA. Emollients such as white soft paraffin, aqueous cream or coconut oil are recommended to counteract dryness because other emollients, for example yellow soft paraffin, may reduce UVB transmission. When atopic dermatitis is treated, continued topical corticosteroid therapy, until this can be reduced due to response to phototherapy or PUVA, is essential.

General ultraviolet safety measures for patients and staff

Patients

- The dose or administered treatment time for every treatment should be checked by at least one trained phototherapist.
- The eyes must be protected with UV-opaque goggles during exposure in the cabinet.
- Patients are advised to avoid additional exposure to UV radiation from direct or artificial sources.
- Male genital protection is recommended because of increased risk of squamous cell cancers with PUVA to this site (although an exception may be made if, for example, genitalia are markedly affected by psoriasis).
- Patients are warned to avoid perfumed products including deodorants and aftershave, as well as topical treatment, except for recommended emollients (for example, aqueous cream or white soft paraffin/liquid paraffin 50:50 mix), prior to treatment.
- The face may be shielded during treatment unless it is affected. A visor (223) or high protection sun barrier preparation can be used.
- When the tubes are changed, do not forget to check the output and adjust the dose table accordingly. If in-built dosimeters are being relied upon, any change in output should be detected automatically and the treatment time altered accordingly. If there have been a number of lamp changes ensure this is the case prior to administering further treatments.

Staff

- Wear protective glasses when you are directly exposed.
- Use screens to protect staff from UV radiation.

Adverse effects of UVB and PUVA

During treatment

Adverse effects are monitored at each visit by asking the patient about any problems following the previous dose, and by examination. The main adverse effect is sunburn-like erythema, which tends to peak at 12–24 hours after UVB and 3–5 days after PUVA, treatments.

- Grade 1: Barely perceptible erythema (224).
- Grade 2: Well-defined erythema compared to shaded sites, for example under arms (225).
- Grade 3: Painful erythema (sometimes called a "burn") (226).

Generalized itch can occur with both PUVA and UVB, although this tends to be more of a problem with PUVA. Frequent application of emollients is usually sufficient to alleviate itch with UVB phototherapy. Some people believe that PUVA itch and PUVA pain, probably caused in some way through PUVA damage to cutaneous nerves, are part of a spectrum. PUVA pain is a serious side effect: it is a severe itch or pain, usually of "burning" or "pins and needles" character, which occurs unpredictably and can last for many months. Topical menthol in aqueous cream, capsaicin cream, oral anxiolytic antihistamines, ultraviolet B phototherapy, and tricyclic antidepressants or anti-epileptics are often tried but all tend to give disappointing results.

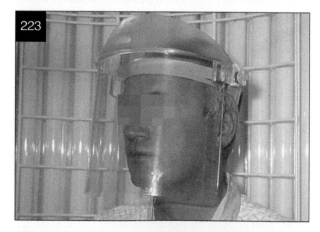

223: A clear UV-absorbing face shield worn to prevent unnecessary exposure of facial skin in a patient with psoriasis of trunk and limbs.

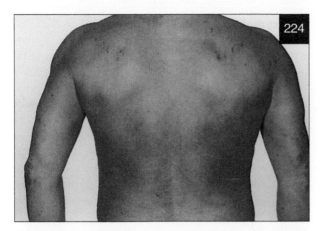

224: Grade I erythema.

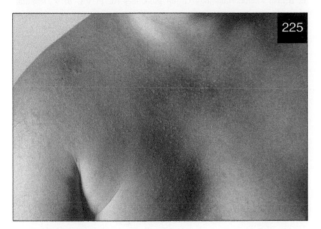

225: Grade 2 erythema.

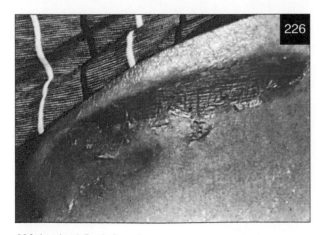

226: Localized Grade 3 erythema.

Polymorphic light eruption is very common and is not infrequently provoked in patients being treated for other conditions such as psoriasis or atopic eczema. Treatment can usually be continued, as for PLE desensitization, with, if necessary, the use of a moderate potency steroid after treatments for symptomatic relief. When PLE occurs for the first time during phototherapy, particularly if severe or persistent, a request for ANF and anti-Ro and La antibodies should be considered to exclude subacute cutaneous lupus erythematosus masquerading as PLE.

The frequency of recurrent herpes labialis is increased but primary infection is not more common. This is presumably due to localized immunosuppression because a sun barrier preparation to the affected site (usually lips) will protect those patients who are prone to this problem.

Chronic

The main chronic adverse effects are skin cancer and photo-aging. The risk of squamous cell carcinoma following PUVA increases with higher cumulative exposures (and cumulative UVA dose). PUVA is also associated with a smaller increased risk of basal cell carcinoma and of melanoma. The risks of broadband UVB exposure have not been well quantified: it is probable that sufficient UVB exposures will also increase a patient's risk of skin cancer. Since the introduction of narrowband UVB in the 1980s, patients have been more carefully followed up so we will eventually know about any late side effects.

It is important that all patients are aware of these risks, so that they know to seek advice about anything that might be a skin cancer. Annual review of at-risk patients (see p.124) is warranted for those who may be at significant risk of these side effects. The purpose of this is to screen for cancerous or precancerous changes, and to remind patients of the need for self-monitoring. Skin cancer risks can be minimized by treating only sites that require it (particularly shielding naturally sunlight-exposed sites from unnecessary exposure), and by keeping cumulative exposures (particularly of PUVA) low. So, treatment courses should be kept as short as possible by following an optimal regimen, maintenance therapy should be avoided unless essential, and concomitant therapy with systemic retinoids should be considered for psoriasis and mycosis fungoides treatment.

However, it should be emphasized that all effective therapies carry risks. Many educated patients with severe psoriasis prefer to accept an increased risk of skin cancer to the risks of alternatives to phototherapy.

Long-term follow-up

It is important to keep a set of phototherapy notes for each patient, recording number of exposures, cumulative dose, and risk factor profile. A computer database system is useful for units treating more than a few patients a year. Patients who have had a large number of exposures (≥150 PUVA exposures or ≥300 UVB treatments), or other significant risk factors (such as past history of skin cancer), should be offered annual review.

New developments

Research into the efficacy of phototherapy in several conditions for which its effectiveness is unconfirmed is ongoing. Also, although several studies have answered questions about how we should administer phototherapy, these have mainly addressed questions relating to the treatment of chronic plaque psoriasis. A lot more research is needed to establish optimal regimens for other conditions: treatment courses will often need to be adjusted for individual patients, but it is useful to have protocols that can be followed for the majority of people with the conditions we treat.

Two fairly recent developments in phototherapy equipment are advances in UVA1 sources and a 308 nm laser. Long-wavelength ultraviolet A (UVA1, 340–400 nm UVA) phototherapy is effective for acute severe atopic dermatitis exacerbations, and is particularly promising as a treatment for conditions such as localized scleroderma and lichen sclerosus (227), for which we do not already have good treatments. High-output UVA1 equipment is bulky and expensive and is currently only available in a few centers. A 308 nm excimer laser capable of treating psoriasis and vitiligo is available. Unless blistering doses are given, it requires multiple treatments, just as does phototherapy with a non-laser source, but where available this treatment may prove useful for the occasional patient with very localized disease for whom conventional whole-body phototherapy, or phototherapy limited to an area such as hands, is not warranted.

Further reading

1. Ibbotson, S.H., et al., An update and guidance on narrowband ultraviolet B phototherapy: a British Photodermatology Group Workshop Report. *Br J Dermatol*, 2004. **151**(2): p. 283-97.

2. Dawe, R.S., Ultraviolet A1 phototherapy. Br J *Dermatol*, 2003. **148**(4): p. 626-37.

3. Dawe, R.S., A quantitative review of studies comparing the efficacy of narrow-band and broad-band ultraviolet B for psoriasis. *Br J Dermatol*, 2003. **149**(3): p. 669-72.

4. Samson Yashar, S., et al., Narrow-band ultraviolet B treatment for vitiligo, pruritus, and inflammatory dermatoses. *Photodermatol Photoimmunol Photomed*, 2003. **19**(4): p. 164-8.

5. Halpern, S.M., et al., Guidelines for topical PUVA: a report of a workshop of the British photodermatology group. Br J Dermatol, 2000. **142**(1): p. 22-31.

6. British Photodermatology Group guidelines for PUVA. *Br J Dermatol*, 1994. **130**(2): p. 246-55.

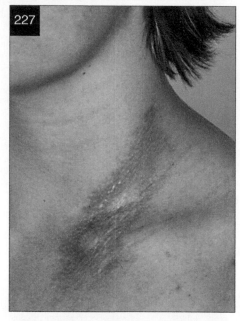

227: Localized morphea over neck. Although this became more noticeable after a course of UVA1 (note the brown pigment, a common UVA1 side effect), the lesion softened and neck mobility improved.

20 Photodynamic Therapy
Sally Ibbotson

History and background

Selective clearance of diseased skin with preservation of normal tissue is the aim of all treatments. Photodynamic therapy (PDT) requires absorption of light of an appropriate wavelength by a photosensitizer in an oxygen-dependent process, resulting in oxidative stress, tissue damage, and cell death. Specificity of treatment is determined by photosensitizer localization and accessibility to light delivery.

Raab first studied the photodynamic effect by investigation of acridine-induced toxicity of protozoa and the demonstration of amplification of toxicity in the presence of daylight.[1] The term "photodynamic reaction" was coined in 1904 and the requirement of oxygen was recognized. Jesionek and Von Tappeiner subsequently reported the beneficial effects of PDT using topical eosin and exposure to sunlight or an arc lamp for the treatment of skin diseases, which included skin cancers and lupus vulgaris.[2]

Investigation of systemic photosensitizers was initiated by Meyer-Betz who demonstrated cutaneous phototoxicity after self-injection with hematoporphyrin and subsequent sun exposure.[3] Silver, in 1937, reported the beneficial effect of intramuscular hematoporphyrin and UV exposure as a treatment for psoriasis.[4] The demonstration of tumor selectivity of porphyrins led to the purification of hematoporphyrin derivative and the pioneering work of Dougherty and colleagues with systemic PDT in patients with a variety of skin tumors.[5] These studies were of fundamental importance in highlighting the potential for PDT as an anticancer therapy. Subsequently, a purified photosensitizer derived from hematoporphyrin, porfimer-sodium (Photofrin), was developed and has approval for use in systemic PDT for several malignancies, including those of lung and esophagus, although it is not approved for dermatologic indications.

Photosensitizers

The properties of an "ideal" photosensitizer include light absorption at clinically useful wavelengths, accumulation in the target tissue, efficiency, and rapid clearance. Several chemicals are under investigation for use in systemic PDT including the porphyrins, porphines, chlorins, phthalocyanines, and texapyrins. Systemic delivery of the porphyrin Photofrin is complicated by visible light photosensitivity for more than 6 weeks (228) and the risk of phototoxicity due to extravasation at injection sites (229). The potent photosensitizer, temoporphin (THPC, Foscan) is under investigation for use in PDT for head and neck cancers and appears to be associated with a

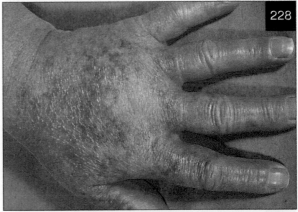

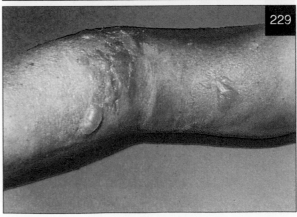

228: Acute phototoxicity, with swelling, erythema and vascular damage on the back of a hand, in a patient after sysemic Photofrin and exposure to trivial amounts of daylight.

229: Acute phototoxicity, with swelling, erythema, and blistering, at the site of Photofrin extravasation in a patient who had undergone systemic PDT.

shorter duration of photosensitivity, and the chlorin benzo-porphyrin derivative-monoacid (BPD-MA, Verteporfin) is used for PDT in macular degeneration.

The skin is accessible and readily targeted by PDT. The prolonged photosensitivity associated with systemically delivered photosensitizers is unacceptable for most patients with skin cancer or skin disease. However, there have been several studies of the use of systemic PDT in the treatment of multiple skin cancers and there may be the potential for use in the treatment of patients with multiple skin tumors, for example in Gorlin syndrome.

The use of a topical photosensitizer would be the ideal approach for PDT in dermatology. Topical application of 5-aminolevulinic acid (ALA) was introduced in 1990 by Kennedy and colleagues and has revolutionized the use of PDT in dermatology;[6] 5-aminolevulinic acid is a precursor in the heme cycle and is not itself a photosensitizer. Topical PDT is now widely used, with application of ALA to the lesion to be treated and subsequent conversion to protoporphyrin IX (PpIX) by the skin cell's heme metabolic pathway (230). The application of exogenous ALA bypasses the negative feedback control and, as the ferrochelatase enzyme is a rate-limiting step, relative accumulation of PpIX occurs in the treated cells. Protoporphyrin IX is a highly efficient endogenous photosensitizer expressed at low concentration in all mammalian nucleated cells but not at levels sufficient to cause photosensitivity.

Systemic ALA has been used in PDT, for example for gastrointestinal malignancies. However, nausea, vomiting, and liver toxicity may occur and limit the use of the systemic route. The principles of tumor selectivity are not fully understood although, after topical application, abnormal permeability of the stratum corneum overlying diseased tissue is a major factor in allowing enhanced penetration of ALA, which is a small hydrophilic molecule. *In vitro* studies suggest that relative iron deficiency, an altered heme enzyme pathway, tumor cell pH, and the state of cell differentiation may be implicated in the relative accumulation of the photosensitizer in diseased tissue. However, selectivity is not specific for neoplastic disease as other benign hyperproliferative conditions, such as viral warts or psoriasis, do show selective PpIX accumulation after ALA application.

There are increasing developments in the use of topical photo-sensitizers in PDT, in particular in the use of lipophilic ALA esters, which may improve photosensitizer uptake and specificity. Protoporphyrin IX is a fluorescent species, which exhibits crimson red fluorescence on Wood's light examination (231, 232). Surface measurements show ratios of up to 15:1 for fluorescence in non-melanoma skin cancer compared with non-lesional skin after a 6-hour ALA application time. Lower ratios are seen using fluorescence microscopy, although in general tumor tissue does show greater accumulation

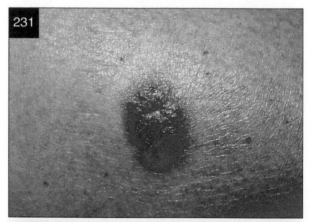

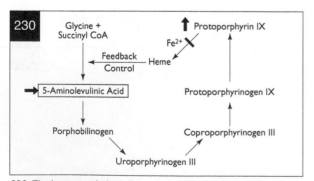

230: The heme metabolic pathway. Bypass of negative feedback control occurs when ALA is applied exogenously (→) and PpIX accumulates (↑) because of the rate-limiting activity of the ferrochelatase enzyme (↓).

231, 232: White light image of superficial basal cell carcinoma (231) and 6 hours after ALA application, crimson red tumor-specific PpIX fluorescence is seen (232).

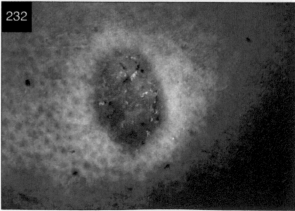

of PpIX than normal skin. A further advantage of ALA PDT is that the photosensitizers formed have a short half-life and prolonged photosensitivity at the treatment site is not a problem, with PpIX clearance by 24–48 h. In an attempt to improve ALA tissue penetration, combination with penetration enhancers or iron chelators such as DMSO, EDTA or desferrioxamine has been investigated, although there is no conclusive evidence for improvement in PDT efficacy. Other photosensitizers are under investigation for potential use in PDT but only topical PDT is discussed for the remainder of this chapter.

Light sources

Most photosensitizers used in PDT absorb maximally in the visible waveband. The absorption spectrum of porphyrins is broad, with peak absorption around 410 nm (Soret band) and additional smaller peaks between 500 and 650 nm (**233**). However, photosensitizer activation needs to occur at the target site, although tissue penetration at 410 nm is poor. Therefore, for topical PDT, light delivery is a compromise, with irradiation around 630–635 nm, improving tissue penetration to a maximum of approximately 6 mm, corresponding with one of the smaller absorption peaks of PpIX. During ALA PDT there is also generation of PpIX photoproducts with absorption peaks around 670 nm.

A range of irradiation sources is available for use in PDT, including monochromatic laser and polychromatic broadband sources, with peak emission in the 630–635 nm waveband. A variety of lasers have been used for PDT including dye lasers pumped by Nd:YAG, copper vapor or argon ion, which were cumbersome and expensive. The use of lasers has been greatly facilitated by the development of cheaper, compact diode lasers, although there is no evidence that they are superior in efficacy to the broadband sources. The latter include a range of commonly used sources: modified slide projector (400–650 nm), tungsten filament halogen lamps (570–680 nm), short arc xenon source with a variable wavelength emission, and metal halide source (600–800 nm), the latter allowing irradiation of fields up to 20 cm in diameter. Each source has advantages and disadvantages, with variables in the field size, irradiance, and treatment times. Exciting new developments with the use of light-emitting diodes (LEDs) indicate that low-output PDT is effective and likely to be an area for further development.

There is wide variation in the light dose and irradiance used in PDT. Irradiation at high intensity reduces treatment times, although animal studies indicate that light delivery at lower irradiance or with fractionation of the dose results in an enhanced photodynamic effect due to tissue re-oxygenation. The importance of tissue oxygenation during PDT is demonstrated by the observation of an enhanced effect with mild hyperthermia and increased oxygen tension in tumor tissue. However, marked hyperthermia results in increased scarring and, in general, infrared wavelengths are excluded during PDT.

Optimal timing of light delivery is essential in order to coincide with the time of peak tissue photosensitizer accumulation. Typically, a 3–6 hour ALA or 3-hour ALA ester application has been used prior to light delivery in topical PDT. Red light is conventionally used, although evidence indicates that either blue or green light ALA PDT is effective for the treatment of actinic keratosis. Photodegradation, "photobleaching" of PpIX, occurs rapidly during irradiation, although some re-accumulation may occur after treatment.

Future photosensitizer developments, with new compounds absorbing maximally in the 700–800 nm wavelength range, with enhanced tissue penetration, may facilitate the treatment of deeper lesions. At present, both photosensitizer and light tissue penetration limit the depth of effective treatment by topical PDT.

Mechanism of action

Most of the evidence relating to the effects of PDT has been derived from studies *in vitro* and, although there appear to be some common molecular events, the effects of PDT depend on the photosensitizer, light delivery, experimental conditions, and cell and tissue type. Important determinants of the PDT effect include the subcellular localization and concentration of the photosensitizer, its activation by light of the appropriate

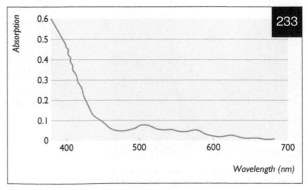

233: The porphyrin absorption spectrum.

wavelength, and the presence of oxygen. Generation of reactive oxygen species, in particular cytotoxic singlet oxygen, occurs with activation of signaling pathways, gene transcription, and cell cycle arrest. PDT may induce apoptosis or necrosis, and membrane, mitochondrial, and nuclear damage may occur. Regulation of cytokines, such as IL-6 and IL-10, and induction of stress response genes, such as heat shock protein and heme oxygenase, may occur and PDT has an immunomodulatory effect. Many of the effects of systemic PDT are mediated by direct involvement of the vasculature, whereas this is thought to be less important for topical PDT. Although PDT has been shown to cause DNA damage, such as strand breaks, and may be mutagenic, there is no evidence for a carcinogenic effect.

Dermatology indications

The main dermatology indications for topical PDT are for the treatment of actinic keratosis, superficial basal cell carcinoma and Bowen's disease. The role of topical PDT in the treatment of other skin diseases is not yet fully defined.

Several treatment options are available for the treatment of actinic keratosis, superficial basal cell carcinoma and Bowen's disease, including surgery, cryotherapy, curettage and cautery, radiotherapy, and 5-fluorouracil, and there is sufficient evidence to include topical PDT as an effective treatment option. In particular, topical PDT should be considered for the treatment of difficult cases, such as multiple lesions of Bowen's disease on the lower legs (234) or multiple truncal basal cell carcinomas (235) or extensive areas of field change actinic keratosis on the scalp. Photodynamic therapy is highly effective in selective cases, it is non-invasive

and well tolerated on an outpatient basis, and repeated treatments are possible. Additionally, in view of its selectivity and tissue-sparing properties, excellent cosmetic results are possible.

Actinic keratosis

Topical ALA PDT has achieved clinical clearance rates of 71–100% for the treatment of actinic keratosis (236). There is variation in methodology, with ALA application times between 3 and 18 hours having been studied and evidence suggesting that a 3–4 hour application period is sufficient. A wide range of irradiation protocols has also been reported. Red and blue light PDT have independently been shown to be effective in the treatment of non-hyperkeratotic actinic keratoses on the face and scalp. However, blue light PDT using a topical solution of ALA (Levulan) applied for 14–18 hours is the only PDT regimen which is approved by the Food and Drug Agency (FDA) for the treatment of actinic keratosis in the USA. In addition, green light PDT has also been shown to be effective in the treatment of actinic keratosis and is less painful than red light PDT. Red light PDT is usually applied for the treatment of actinic keratosis in Europe, with light doses generally of the order of 100–150 J/cm² and, although a single treatment is usually sufficient, a second may be necessary. Acral and hypertrophic actinic keratoses respond less well to PDT (30–45% complete response), although equivalent efficacy to 5-fluorouracil has been demonstrated in a comparative study. Two studies compared methyl ester ALA PDT with cryotherapy for the treatment of actinic keratosis, mainly on the face and scalp, one showing equivalent efficacy at 3 months but improved cosmetic outcome after PDT and the other showing superior efficacy and cosmetic outcome following PDT. Indeed, topical PDT with ALA methyl ester and red light is now approved in Europe for the treatment

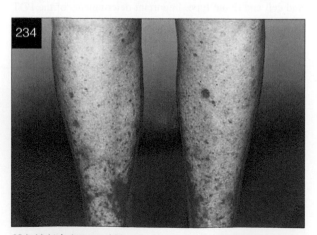

234: Multiple lesions of Bowen's disease and actinic keratoses on the lower legs of an elderly woman ideally suited for topical PDT.

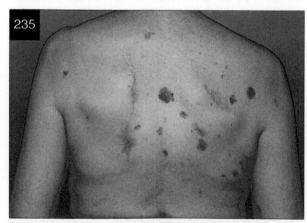

235: Multiple superficial basal cell carcinomas on the trunk of an elderly patient ideally suited for topical PDT. Note the previous scars from surgery.

of non-hypertrophic actinic keratosis on the face and scalp.

So to summarize, ALA PDT and methyl ester ALA PDT are effective in the treatment of actinic keratosis, particularly for non-hyperkeratotic lesions on the face and scalp, with efficacy at least equivalent to 5-fluorouracil and cryotherapy, but with improved cosmetic results. Topical PDT appears to be an ideal treatment option for widespread thin actinic keratoses, such as on the head and neck.

Bowen's disease

Complete response rates of up to 100% have been reported for the treatment of Bowen's disease by systemic PDT, although the side effect of prolonged photosensitivity precludes its routine use. Several open and randomized comparative studies have been performed showing 85–100% clearance rates with one or two ALA PDT treatments for Bowen disease (**237**). The recurrence rates average 12% over follow-up periods of up to 36 months. In two separate randomized studies, topical ALA PDT was compared with cryotherapy and 5-fluorouracil, showing PDT to be at least as effective as cryotherapy and superior to 5-fluorouracil, but associated with fewer side effects. A variety of treatment regimens have been used, although typically ALA applications of 3–6 hours have been used and irradiation protocols using laser or broadband sources and light doses generally in the range of 100–150 J/cm². Red light PDT has been shown to be superior to green light PDT in the treatment of Bowen's disease, showing both a higher clearance rate and lower incidence of recurrence. The use of ALA ester PDT may improve efficacy in the treatment of Bowen's disease and with excellent cosmetic outcome, although comparative studies with ALA have not been performed. Topical PDT is highly effective and ideal for the treatment of large or multiple patches of Bowen's disease, particularly those at difficult body sites (**238**) and sites of poor healing, such as the lower leg.

Superficial basal cell carcinoma

Systemic PDT has shown high rates of clearance for the treatment of basal cell carcinoma, although with recurrence rates of up to almost 50%. For ALA PDT, initial clearance rates of 80–100% are reported with one or two treatments for superficial

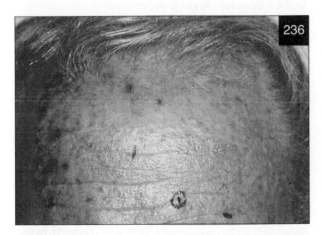

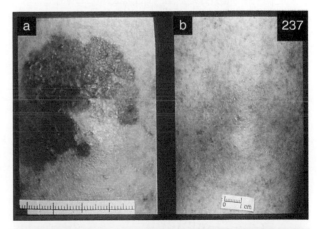

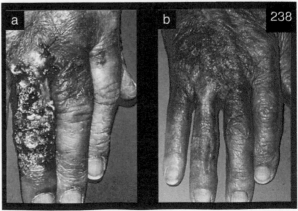

236: Actinic keratoses on the forehead of an elderly male of skin type I 3 months after treatment of the left half of the forehead with a single treatment of topical ALA PDT.

237: (a) Bowen's disease on the lower leg of an elderly patient and (b) clinical response 3 months after a single treatment with topical ALA PDT.

238: (a) Neglected Bowen's disease on the finger of an elderly male and (b) clearance after two treatments with topical ALA PDT.

basal cell carcinoma (**239, 240**), with recurrence rates of up to 18% over 24 months documented. An increased ALA application time from 4 to 6 hours is required for clearance of tumors up to 2 mm in thickness, with 100% response documented in a small study and no recurrence up to 16 months. Several irradiation regimens have been used with wide variation in light doses, although it appears that a dose of at least 75 J/cm² may be required and that laser and non-laser sources are of equivalent efficacy.

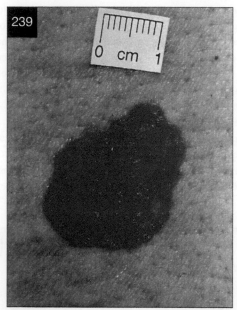

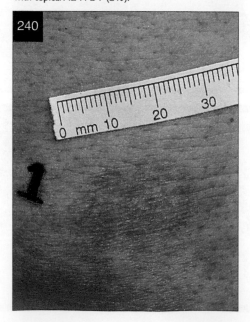

239, 240: Superficial basal cell carcinoma on the trunk (239) and clearance 3 months after a single treatment with topical ALA PDT (240).

Nodular basal cell carcinomas respond less well to topical PDT, which is considered to be due to lack of homogenous PpIX accumulation and poor light penetration. Initial curettage and use of penetration enhancers or iron chelators, such as DMSO and EDTA, can achieve response rates of up to 95% and the use of ALA esters may improve these results further. Photodynamic therapy has been shown to be at least as effective as cryotherapy for superficial basal cell carcinoma but with fewer side effects and improved cosmesis, and two treatments 7 days apart may improve response rates. Large or multiple truncal or lower leg superficial basal cell carcinomas or lesions at cosmetically difficult sites (**241, 242**) are ideally suited for PDT.

A recent report by the British Photodermatology Group recommended PDT as an effective treatment for superficial basal cell carcinomas less than 2 mm in thickness, although it is not suitable for nodular basal cell carcinoma unless combined with curettage or penetration enhancers. Superior outcomes may be achieved using ALA esters. Topical PDT with ALA methyl ester and red light is now approved for the treatment of superficial basal cell carcinoma in Europe.

Other dermatologic indications

Randomized, controlled, and comparative studies are available, indicating that ALA PDT is effective in the treatment of selected cases of recalcitrant *viral warts* (**243, 244**). ALA PDT has additionally been shown to be effective in the treatment of both truncal and facial acne, with response maintained over several months. The use of ALA PDT in *psoriasis* has been studied with disappointing results, showing a lack of homogenous photosensitizer accumulation in psoriatic plaque and unpredictable and painful treatment responses. Preliminary evidence indicates that topical PDT may be of use in the treatment of *cutaneous Tcell lymphoma*, although further studies are required. The remaining literature relates to the use of topical PDT in case series or case reports for the treatment of several skin diseases *(Table 20.1)*. However, further work is required to substantiate the role of PDT in the management of these conditions.

Poor response to topical PDT

Lesions that do not respond well to topical PDT include nodular basal cell carcinoma and pigmented tumors, such as pigmented basal cell carcinomas or malignant melanoma, in view of the absorption of red light by melanin. Morpheic basal cell carcinomas do not fluoresce or respond well after ALA application and PDT. Despite efficacy in response of early squamous cell carcinoma to PDT, there is an unacceptably high recurrence rate and PDT is not the treatment of choice. Subcutaneous metastases, for example breast carcinoma, do not respond well to topical PDT with existing regimens, although improved responses have been reported with systemic PDT.

Methodology

Histologic diagnosis should be obtained prior to PDT and, if several lesions are present, biopsies from representative lesions should be taken. If lesions are markedly hyperkeratotic

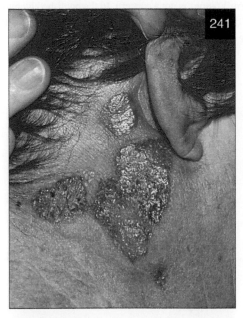

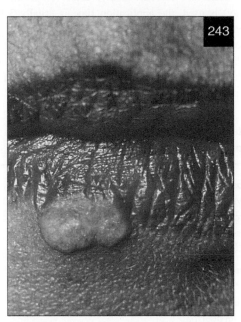

241, 242: Extensive superficial basal cell carcinoma on the neck at a cosmetically difficult site (241) and almost complete clearance after two topical ALA PDT treatments. One small focus of disease remained and was retreated (242).

243, 244: A recalcitrant viral wart on the lower lip before (243) and after (244) three treatments with topical ALA PDT.

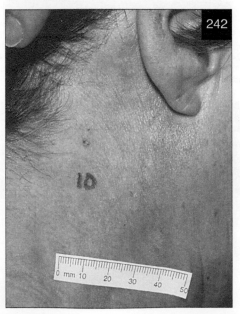

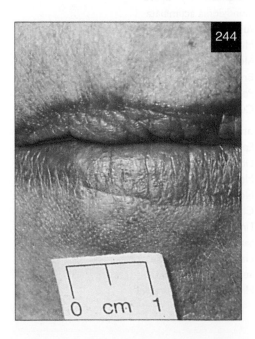

or crusted, gentle surface preparation without local anesthesia using a spatula or curette is advised, in order to facilitate ALA uptake. Application of ALA (in oil-in-water vehicle; for example 20% in Unguentum M, (Crawfords Pharmaceuticals, UK) to the lesion for 4 (actinic keratosis, Bowen's disease) or 6 (superficial basal cell carcinoma) hours is performed under occlusion. If ALA-methyl ester (Photocure ASA, Norway) is used, the application time is usually 3 hours. Lesions on photo-exposed sites should be covered with a light-opaque dressing to prevent initiation of a PDT effect and photobleaching of PpIX. Photosensitization at the treatment site may last for 24–48 hours and patients should be advised to photoprotect the treated site during this period.

After ALA or ALA ester application (**245**) the dressing is removed and the cream wiped from the area. Wood's light examination should be performed in order to confirm the presence of tissue localized PpIX fluorescence (**231, 232**). Irradiation (**246**) should be performed with a rim of normal tissue included (approximately 5 mm) and, as low levels of PpIX accumulation in normal tissues are rapidly photobleached by irradiation, toxicity to normal tissues is not a concern. In the published literature, the light doses used in PDT vary widely, although typically are of the order of 75–150 J/cm².

Table 20.1: Non-NMSC skin diseases in which topical PDT has been applied

Most studied
• Warts
• Acne
• Psoriasis
• Cutaneous T cell lymphoma

Case series
• Actinic cheilitis and leukoplakia
• Keratoacanthoma
• Scleroderma
• Lichen sclerosus
• Erythroplasia of Queyrat
• Extramammary Paget's
• Condyloma acuminata
• Vulval intra-epithelial neoplasia
• Hirsutism
• Alopecia areata
• Breast metastases
• Porokeratosis
• Cutaneous leishmaniasis

Case reports
• Epidermodysplasia verruciformis
• Lichen planus
• Melanoma
• Nevus sebaceous
• Chondrodermatitis nodularis helicis
• Tinea pedis
• Sarcoid
• Hailey–Hailey disease
• Sebaceous hyperplasia
• Hidradenitis suppurativa

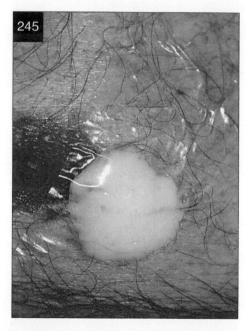

245, 246: ALA (20% in Ung MI is applied under occlusion for 4 hours (actinic keratosis, Bowen's disease) or 6 hours (superficial basal cell carcinoma) (245) and then irradiation is performed(246).

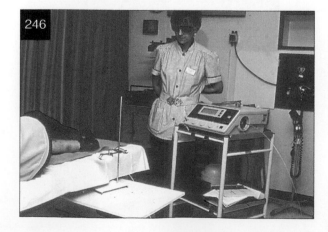

Adverse effects of PDT

Patients having undergone systemic PDT require visible light photoprotection with behavioral modification, clothing cover, and the use of physical sunscreens with visible light protection for up to approximately 3 months or more after treatment. Cautious daylight exposure is required in order for photodegradation of residual cutaneous photosensitizer to occur. Topical PDT is usually well tolerated, although both acute and chronic adverse effects can occur. It is usual to expect minor pain, burning, and tingling at the site during irradiation, and indeed a prickling sensation may be apparent even with ALA application alone.

The majority of PDT treatments can be performed without local anesthesia. However, in our experience, up to 19% of patients find treatment extremely painful and this does appear to be related to the use of high-intensity irradiation sources, such as laser light delivery. A cooling fan or cold air and lignocaine spray during irradiation may alleviate discomfort and, if a large area requires treatment, topical local anesthesia using either EMLA or amethocaine (Ametop), or the use of injectable plain lignocaine, should be considered, although they may offer only minor pain relief. The mechanisms of pain are not well defined and patients commonly find the discomfort most severe in the first few minutes of treatment, with subsequent reduction in the symptoms experienced. Fractionation of the irradiation dose may also be of benefit in terms of pain reduction.

Following PDT, an immediate erythemal reaction is to be expected and edema at the treatment site may occur, with urticaria in a minority (**247, 248**). The phototoxicity of PDT in normal skin is most apparent within 1 hour after exposure and subsequently reduces and resolves over a 4–5 day period. There is inter-individual variation in phototoxicity after topical PDT in normal skin and in erythemal sensitivity depending on body site and irradiation source. A crust usually forms at the treatment site over a week or two before separating off, and pigmentary change may occur in a minority (**249, 250**),

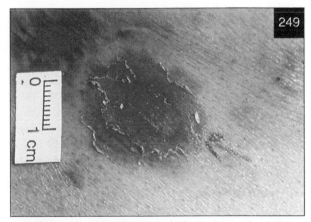

247, 248: An acute erythemal response is expected immediately after topical ALA PDT (247) and some patients develop edema and urticaria at the treatment site (248).

249, 250: Although uncommon, both hyperpigmentation (249) and hypopigmentation (250) can occur, although both are usually temporary.

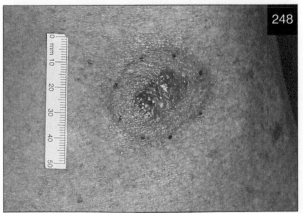

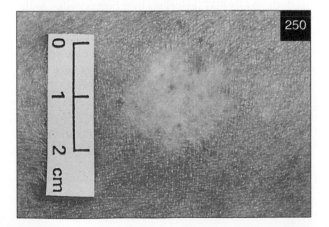

although this generally resolves with time. Ulceration of the treatment site is a rare occurrence and absent or minimal scarring is evident after treatment. There appear to be no significant long-term risks of PDT and, although the development of a melanoma on the scalp of a patient treated with topical PDT is of concern, this appears to have been an isolated and coincidental event. To date there is no evidence for carcinogenicity of PDT.

Fluorescence diagnosis

The fluorescence of PpIX may be applied diagnostically and therapeutically, for example to monitor the efficacy of PDT, to investigate the rate of recovery of PpIX after PDT using real-time *in vivo* fluorescence measurements, and to delineate surgical excision margins for ill-defined tumors. Fluorescence diagnosis is an exciting area of development with considerable potential clinical impact.

Conclusions and future developments

Topical PDT is established as an effective therapy for the treatment of actinic keratosis, Bowen's disease, and superficial basal cell carcinoma. Studies indicate similar or superior efficacy of PDT compared with conventional treatments for these conditions, with reduced adverse effects and superior cosmetic outcome for PDT. Further developments in photosensitizers and their delivery, such as the ALA esters and the use of penetration enhancers, will refine the use of topical PDT. The future development of systemic photosensitizers with high safety profiles and minimal generalized photosensitivity may facilitate the use of systemic PDT in the treatment of patients with multiple lesions or, for example, conditions such as psoriasis. There is a need for standardization of the methodology for PDT (guidelines have been published by the British Photodermatology Group) and for further consideration of the methods of light delivery. Studies are also required with respect to investigating the molecular effects of PDT, the pain of PDT, and the optimization of treatment of thicker basal cell carcinomas and other skin diseases. Finally, the area of fluorescence diagnosis is likely to have increasing clinical impact and is one of several areas of development, which highlights the expanding role of PDT in dermatology.

References

1. Raab O. Uber die Wirkung flourescierender Stoffe auf Infusoria. *Z Biol* 1900; **39**: 524.

2. Jesionek A, Von Tappeiner H. Zur Behandlung de Hautcarcinome mit fl"uoreszierenden Stoffen. *Dtsch Arch Klin Med* 1905; **85**: 223-39.

3. Meyer-Betz F. Untersuchungen uber die biologische (photodynamische) Wirkung des Hamatopotphyrins und andere Derivate des Blut- und Gallenfarbstoffes. *Dtsch Arch Klin Med* 1913;**112**:476-503.

4 Silver H. Psoriasis vulgaris treated with hematoporphyrin. *Arch Dermatol Syph* 1937; **36**: 1118-19.

5. Dougherty TJ, Kaufman JE, Goldfarb A, Weishaupt KR, Boyle D, Mittleman A. Photoradiation therapy for the treatment of malignant tumors. *Cancer Res* 1978;**38**: 2628–35.

6. Kennedy JC, Pottier RH, Pross DC. Photodynamic therapy with endogenous protoporphyrin IX: basic principles and present clinical experience. *J Photochem Photobiol, B: Biol* 1990;**6**:143–8.

Further reading

Brancaleon L, Moseley H. Lasers and non-laser light sources for photodynamic therapy. *Lasers Med Sci* 2002;**17**:173–86.

Dragieva G, Prinz BM, Hafner J, Burg G, Binswanger U, Kempf W. A randomised controlled clinical trial of topical photodynamic therapy with methyl aminolaevulinate in the treatment of actinic keratosis in transplant recipients. *Br J Dermatol* 2004; **151**: 196-200

Fritsch C, Goerz G, Ruzicka T. Photodynamic therapy in dermatology. *Arch Dermatol* 1998;**134**:207–14.

Ibbotson SH.Topical 5-aminolaevulinic acid photodynamic therapy for the treatment of skin conditions other than non-melanoma skin cancer. *Br J Dermatol* 2002;**146**:178–88.

Kalka K, Merk H, Mukhtar H. Photodynamic therapy in dermatology. *J Am Acad Dermatol* 2000;**42**:389–413.

Morton CA, Brown SB, Collins S et al. Guidelines for topical photodynamic therapy: a report of a workshop of the British Photodermatology Group. *Br J Dermatol* 2002;**146**:552–67.

Peng Q, Berg K, Moan J, Kongshaug M, Nesland JM. 5-aminolevulinic acid-based photodynamic therapy: principles and experimental research. *Photochem Photobiol* 1997;**65**:235`-51.

Peng Q, Warloe T, Berg K et al. 5-aminolevulinic acid-based photodynamic therapy. Clinical research and future challenges. *Cancer* 1997;**79**:2282–308.

Varma S, Wilson H, Kurwa HA et al. Bowen's disease, solar keratoses and superficial basal cell carcinomas treated by photodynamic therapy using a large-field incoherent light source. *Br J Dermatol* 2001;**144**:567–74.

Pollock B, Turner D, Stringer MR, Bojar RA, Goulden V, Stables GI, Cunliffe WJ. Topical aminolaevulinic acid-photodynamic therapy for the treatment of acne vulgaris: a study of clinical efficacy and mechanism of action. *Br J Dermatol* 2004; **151**: 616-622

21 Laser–tissue Interactions

Harry Moseley

Principles of laser generation

The term "laser" was coined as an acronym for light amplification by stimulated emission of radiation, which describes the principle of operation of the device. Although Albert Einstein first postulated the theorem governing stimulated emission in 1917, it was not until 1960 that Theodore Maiman demonstrated the first practical laser – the ruby laser.

Strictly speaking the term "laser" describes the process of production and amplification of light. Atoms and molecules exist within well-defined energy bands. Transition from a higher energy to a lower energy band is accompanied by emission of radiation. This occurs naturally and produces spontaneous emission. By contrast, within a laser, excited atoms and molecules are stimulated to release radiation by the action of an incident photon having precisely the same energy as the gap in the atomic energy level. The stimulated radiation photon has the same wavelength as the incident photon, is exactly in phase with it, and both photons move off in the same direction (**251**).

In this process there is amplification of light, since two identical photons emerge from the atoms. Moreover, these photons continue to interact with other excited atoms to produce yet more photons – and further light amplification. For this to happen, it is necessary to create what is known as a population inversion. Normally, atoms and molecules exist in the lowest energy states possible. For lasing action to take place, there must be an increase in the number of atoms in an excited energy state. This requires energy to continuously pump atoms into higher energy states. In addition, the ends of the laser cavity are highly reflective so that the photons are reflected back into the lasing material many times. One end is partially reflective, allowing some of the stimulated radiation to emerge through a small aperture. This is the laser beam.

All lasers have a common basic configuration that is necessary for the production of stimulated emission of radiation. The source of excitation energy generates the excited species within the laser medium. Mirrors define the laser cavity (or resonator). A partially reflecting mirror permits a small fraction of the radiation within the cavity to leave so as to maintain a high photon density in the laser medium to sustain the stimulated emission (**252**).

Many spontaneous and stimulated photons will be lost through the sides of the laser cavity. However, those which

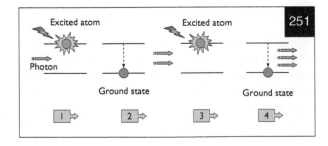

251: Diagram of stimulated emission.

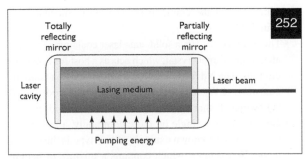

252: Components of a laser.

travel along the axis of the cavity will be reflected off the end-mirrors, all the time stimulating more photons. This results in a very high concentration of identical photons moving in parallel along the axis of the laser cavity.

The lasing medium may be gas (for example, argon), liquid (for example, organic dye), or solid (for example, ruby crystal). The pumping energy may be light or an electric discharge. If the laser is excited by a single burst of energy, the output will be pulsed but if, on the other hand, the laser is pumped continuously, this will produce a continuous wave (CW) laser emission.

Properties of laser light

Laser light has unique properties that make it extremely useful in medicine (253).

- *Monochromatic laser light* has a very narrow bandwidth. Most lasers are actually able to emit more than a single wavelength but are usually constructed so that only one wavelength is emitted. This means that a laser has excellent spectral purity.
- In *collimated laser light* the beam emerges from the laser cavity as a narrow pencil of light with very little divergence. This means it can be transmitted at extremely high density over considerable distances. If the beam is transmitted down a fiber, it is no longer collimated.
- In *coherent laser light* the wavefront is in phase in time and space. This contrasts with ordinary light, where random emission occurs in all directions, resulting in incoherent light.

Laser radiation may have very high irradiance because of the small cross-sectional area.

$$100\,W \text{ over } 1\,mm^2 = 10,000\,W/cm^2$$

Laser types

Lasers are named according to the lasing material they contain. Some of the common lasers used in medicine are listed in *Table 21.1*.

- The *Nd:YAG laser* is a solid-state laser containing yttrium-alumimum-garnet crystal, which acts as a host for neodymium ions. The Nd:YAG laser operates either as a continuous wave (CW) long pulsed device or in a mode called "Q-switched" that emits very short (nanosecond) pulses.
- *Gas lasers* use a single or, more commonly, a mixture of gases. The best known example of this type is the *helium neon (HeNe) laser*, which contains a mixture of helium and neon gas as the lasing medium, and emits at 632 nm

in the visible red spectrum. It is most commonly used as a pointer and also, superimposed onto the path of invisible infrared lasers, as an aiming beam. Nowadays, the semiconductor diode laser (described below) has replaced the HeNe in many applications. Other gas lasers include the *CO_2 laser* emitting at 10.6 µm, *argon* and *krypton*, emitting at various lines within the visible region.

- *Dye lasers* use organic dyes as the lasing medium and are characterized by their "tunability". A broad range of wavelengths at or near the visible region is possible, depending on the dye used and its concentration.
- *Semiconductor diode lasers* are now in widespread use in medicine and elsewhere. Although they emit at relatively low power, they are built as arrays in order to provide sufficient power for clinical use. Despite this construction, they are physically very small, portable, and cheap. They are available over a wide range of wavelengths, chiefly in the near infrared.

Photochemical effects

The nature of the reaction between the laser beam and tissue depends on many factors including laser wavelength, irradiance, exposure duration and beam diameter, and tissue optical and thermal characteristics. Photochemical effects are seen when the laser wavelength matches the absorption characteristics of some chromophore contained within the tissue and produces a chemical response with no discernible temperature rise. This may occur at low levels of irradiance. The chromophore may be endogenous or exogenous. An example of the former is the photochemical reaction that occurs in the retina on exposure to light. The eye is particularly sensitive to blue light and laser users are cautioned against prolonged exposure to blue light. A common example of the use of an exogenous chromophore is photodynamic therapy (PDT), a technique whereby a tumor is sensitized to light by a photo-active drug.

Photothermal effects

Most applications of lasers in medicine rely on the photothermal effect; that is to say, it is the conversion of energy into heat that is responsible for the tissue response. The thermal effect has several components (254). As the temperature rises beyond approximately 55°C, the tissue is damaged due to denaturation of protein and coagulation, invoking an inflammatory response. This may cause a coagulative necrosis with tissue sloughing off over the following few days. This coagulative effect is useful for sealing blood vessels. Tissue blanching and contraction are also observed. The Nd:YAG laser has very good coagulative properties caused by the fact that the beam penetrates down to 7 mm or 8 mm of tissue (**255**). This means that the radiant power is absorbed within a fairly large volume of tissue and hence the temperature rise is relatively low.

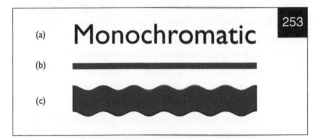

253: Laser radiation is (a) monochromatic, (b) collimated, and (c) coherent.

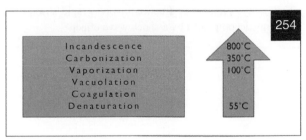

254: Thermal effects of lasers on tissue.

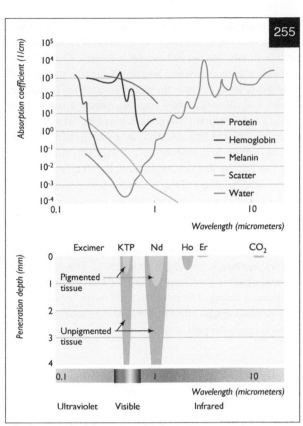

255: Absorption of radiation energy by various chromophores and water in tissue (courtesy Lumenis).

Table 21.1: **Characteristics of lasers commonly used in dermatology**

Laser type	Wavelength (nm)	Power/energy	Duration	Chromophore
Excimer (ArF)	193	0.1 J	20 ns	Protein
Argon	488, 514	3–10 W	0.1-10 s	Hemoglobin
KTP	532	15 W	10 ms	Hemoglobin
Dye (flashlamp-pumped)	577, 585, 595	15 J	1.5 ms	Hemoglobin
Ruby (Q-switched)	694	3 J	25 ns	Tattoos, melanin
Alexandrite	755	50 J	10 ms	Melanin
Alexandrite (Q-switched)	755	10 J	50 ns	Tattoos
Nd:YAG (Q-switched)	1,064	20 mJ	10 ns	Tattoos, protein
Er:YAG	2,940	2 J	500 μs	Protein, water
CO_2	10,600	100 W	1.4 ms	Water

As the temperature continues to rise, both intra- and extracellular water boils at 100°C, and water vapor is formed. As this happens, cellular debris flies out and a crater is formed. The CO_2 laser is highly absorbed by water. As a result, the penetration depth is of the order of 0.1 mm. So all the laser power is absorbed within a small volume of tissue. Vaporization is clearly of value for destruction of large tumor masses. Also, the CO_2 laser can be used like a scalpel, as a cutting tool. To some extent, cutting and coagulation are mutually exclusive. In order to achieve thermal coagulation, the CO_2 laser beam is defocused. The effect of this is that the laser power is spread over a larger area, thereby reducing the intensity so that there is insufficient intensity to cause vaporization.

With sustained exposure, tissue temperature continues to rise rapidly, resulting in charring at about 350°C. This is blackened carbon, which is often seen lining the crater. Furthermore, as the beam is absorbed by this blackened tissue, incandescence may be observed, an effect that may also be seen when tissue particles cross the path of the beam.

Selective photothermolysis

The concept of selective photothermolysis was first postulated by Anderson and Parrish.[1] Prior to this, it was well known that the wavelength of the laser should match the absorption peak of the chromophore. To this was now added the need to select a pulse of suitable duration, depending on the size of the absorbing substance (256). The elements necessary to achieve selective photothermolysis are as follows.
- A unique structure that acts as a target within the lesion to be treated.
- A wavelength that is selectively absorbed by the structure.
- A pulse duration that matches the thermal relaxation of the target.
- Sufficient energy delivered during exposure to damage the lesion.

Thermal relaxation time (TRT) is the time required for an object to cool to 50% of its temperature immediately following laser exposure. If the pulse duration is too short, the object will not be heated up sufficiently throughout its entirety. On the other hand, if the pulse duration is too long, then much of the heat will be conducted to adjacent structures, resulting in collateral damage. For capillaries of diameter 5 μm, TRT is 25 μs; for small venules of diameter 20 μm, TRT is 400 μs; for large ectatic vessels (as in PWS) of diameter 0.1 mm, TRT is 10 ms. For tattoo pigment granules TRT is of the order of 10–100 ns.

Photomechanical effects

Photomechanical effects require a very high-power, short-duration laser pulse. Typically, power density is of the order of 10^{16} W/m^2 or 1 trillion watts per square centimeter, and exposure time is about 1 ns. This is described as a non-linear process which means that doubling the laser power does not double the mechanical effect. There is a threshold power density below which mechanical effects are not observed. At sufficiently high power densities, electrons are stripped from the absorbing medium and this produces a state of ionized matter known as a plasma. The collapse of the plasma produces a shock wave which is dissipated in the surrounding tissue and causes disruption to nearby structures. This contrasts with a photothermal effect where tissue temperature is raised (257). Associated with the collapse of the electrical plasma, there is often a flash of white light and an audible crack. The mechanism of tattoo dye pigment destruction involves rapid absorption of energy accompanied by a shock wave effect.

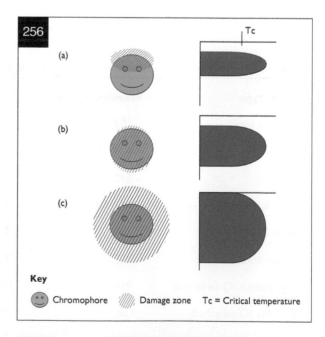

256: Diagram demonstrating effect of pulse duration: (a) pulse duration too short; (b) pulse duration ~ thermal relaxation time; (c) pulse duration too long.

Photo-ablative effects

Photo-ablation is a process whereby a laser beam breaks molecular bonds (**258**). To achieve this, a high photon energy is required. This necessitates the use of excimer lasers that operate in the short wavelength UV region. Photo-ablation is an extremely precise technique and is used to reshape the cornea correction of vision. The technique relies on the laser beam breaking molecular bonds within the cornea with little or no rise in temperature. Lasers operating at a wavelength of 193 nm have been widely used in this procedure. Photon energy at 193 nm is 6.4 eV, which is enough to cleave peptide bonds or adjacent carbon bonds. Ablation of the cornea at 193 nm causes a damage zone of only 0.1–0.3 µm.

Laser safety

The eye is the target site for damage. The nature of the hazard depends on the wavelength, irradiance, exposure duration, spot size, and directional properties of the laser beam. A recent study has shown that operator error was the key factor contributing to medical laser accidents.[3]

The wavelength determines the tissue at risk within the eye. Short wavelength ultraviolet radiation (UVB and UVC) is absorbed by the cornea and, therefore, represents a threat to corneal tissue. Longer wavelength (UVA) is principally absorbed by the intra-ocular crystalline lens and prolonged exposure may induce cataract formation. Light in the visible and near infrared region (400–1400 nm) is transmitted to the retina and so this constitutes the most seriously damaging wavelength region. In contrast to corneal damage, a retinal burn is permanent and cannot be repaired surgically. Consequently, particular care must be exercised when using lasers such as argon, KTP, alexandrite, dye, Nd:YAG, and diode. At longer wavelengths (for example, CO_2 laser), the beam is absorbed in the cornea.

The smallest spot size is obtained by focusing a parallel beam of light. A collimated beam incident on the cornea can undergo four orders of magnitude increase in irradiance as it is focused on to the retina. For example, a beam of 50 W/m^2 on the cornea becomes a 5 MW/m^2 beam on the retina, with a massive increase in damage potential.

Within the eye, it is the fovea at the center of the macula that is responsible for central vision. If laser light is incident on this region the individual is likely to sustain permanent and serious damage, with loss of central vision in that eye. A simple but essential message is: never look directly at the laser beam.

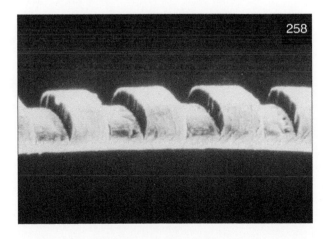

257: Photothermal effect (upper): continuous exposure of match head to laser beam causing temperature rise. Photomechanical effect (lower): short exposure causing ablative pitting of match head.
258: 50 µm notches etched in human hair with an excimer laser.

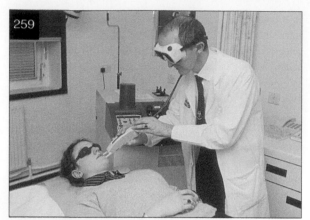

259: Eye goggles should be worn when the laser is in use.

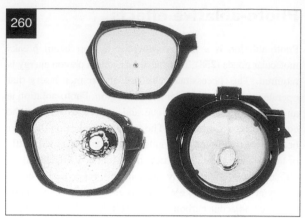

260: Laser goggles subject to burn-through following deliberate exposure to a medical laser beam.[3]

The laser operator and assistants should use protective eyewear **(259)**. This should be selected taking account of the laser wavelength (since absorption is strongly wavelength dependent), comfort, optical density, and damage threshold. This last point is important because protective eyewear may be damaged by direct exposure to the laser beam **(260)**.

In contrast to the eye, accidental laser exposure of the skin is much less damaging although it may cause a painful burn.

Clearly the patient is also at risk from accidental exposure to the laser beam. One of the greatest concerns is that of endotracheal tube ignition when laser surgery is being performed in the vicinity of an ET tube. Such incidents have occurred with fatal consequences.[2]

Other less serious problems may occur. If the skin has been cleaned using an alcohol-based preparation, it is essential that the alcohol vapor has evaporated completely or this may be ignited.

The patient's eyes should be protected at all times. If laser procedures are being carried out in close proximity to the eye, a laser-proof contact lens should be used.

References

1. Anderson RR, Parrish JA. Selective photothermolysis: precise microsurgery by selective absorption of pulsed radiation. *Science* 1983;**220**:524–7.

2. Cozine K. Laser-induced endotracheal tube fire. *Anesthesiology* 1981;**55**:585.

3. Moseley H. Operator error is the key factor contributing to medical laser accidents. *Lasers in Medical Science* **19**:105-111, 2004

4. Fenner J, Moseley H. Damage thresholds of CO_2 laser protective eyewear. *Lasers Med Sci* 1989;**4**:33–9.

Further reading

Lanigan SW. *Lasers in Dermatology.* London: Springer, 2000.

Lask GP, Lowe NJ, eds. *Lasers in Cutaneous and Cosmetic Surgery.* Philadelphia: Churchill Livingstone, 2000.

22 Laser Therapy for Vascular Lesions

Alexander J Stratigos and Jeffrey S Dover

A variety of lasers have been used for the treatment of congenital and acquired vascular lesions. The development of the pulsed dye laser (PDL, 585 nm) based on the principles of selective photothermolysis redefined the therapy of vascular disorders, particularly of hemangiomas, port-wine stains, and telangiectasias.[1] The addition of lasers with longer wavelengths, longer pulse durations and higher energy fluences in conjunction with active epidermal cooling has significantly enhanced our ability to treat vascular lesions.

Types of lasers used for vascular lesions

The lasers used for vascular lesions are separated into two main groups: pulsed lasers and continuous wave (CW) and quasi-continuous wave lasers. The latter group includes the argon laser (488, 514 nm), the argon pumped tunable dye laser (488–638 nm), the potassium titanyl phosphate or KTP laser (532 nm), the krypton laser (568 nm), and the copper vapor and copper bromide lasers (578 nm). Because of the extensive thermal diffusion induced by CW and quasi-CW lasers, the risk of adverse effects is quite high and their use has been limited to selected cases, such as nodular PWS, high-flow spider angiomas, pyogenic granulomas, and thick venous lakes. The pulsed lasers and light sources include the pulsed dye lasers, the pulsed KTP lasers, the pulsed infrared lasers and the intense pulsed light source (Table 22.1).

Pulsed dye laser

The flashlamp-pumped pulsed dye laser (PDL) uses a high-power flashlamp to energize an organic dye (rhodamine) and produce a true pulse of yellow light at 585 nm.[2] Conforming to the principles of selective photothermolysis, the 450 μs pulse duration of the original PDL is shorter than the calculated thermal relaxation time of cutaneous vasculature (1–3 ms for vessel diameter of 10 and 100 μm respectively), allowing for sufficient energy absorption by oxyhemoglobin to cause red blood cell coagulation. The classic PDL is considered to be the treatment of choice for many vascular lesions, such as port-wine stains, particularly in young infants and children, facial telangiectasia including spider angiomas and telangiectatic erythema associated with rosacea, superficial hemangiomas, and poikiloderma of Civatte.

Long-pulsed dye lasers

Recently long-pulsed dye lasers with deeper penetrating wavelengths (595 and 600 nm) and extended pulse durations (1.5 up to 40 ms) have been developed that heat the vessels more gently and produce less profound and less long-lasting purpura than the original PDL. Choices of fluence and pulse duration that induce purpura remain more effective at lightening PWS than long pulse durations that produce sub-purpura treatment. The latter are, however, effective in improving facial redness and some visible facial vessels without producing purpura and thus are distinctly advantageous in the clinical setting.[3] The addition of active cooling systems,

Table 22.1: Pulsed lasers and light sources for vascular lesions

Laser type	Wavelength (nm)	Pulse duration
Pulsed KTP laser	532	1–200 ms
Pulsed dye	585	450 μs
Long-pulsed dye	590, 595, 600	1.5 ms
Variable pulsed dye	600	0.5–40 ms
Long-pulsed alexandrite	755	3–20 ms
Diode	800, 810, 930	1–1000 ms
Long-pulsed Nd:YAG	1064	1–500 ms
Intense pulsed light source	515–1200	0.5–20 ms

such as cryogen spray or air cooling systems has further improved the efficacy of these lasers by allowing the safe delivery of much higher energy fluences for the treatment of resistant vascular lesions, while simultaneously reducing the pain and discomfort associated with laser therapy.

Pulsed KTP lasers

Long-pulse frequency-doubled Nd:YAG or KTP lasers emitting green light at 532 nm have been developed with a specific aim to treat vascular anomalies, particularly facial telangiectasia, without postoperative purpura.[4] The distinct advantage of this group of lasers is the strong absorption of their wavelength by hemoglobin and the longer pulse durations (1–100 ms) that thermally damage the vessels without causing rupture and purpura.

Long-pulsed infrared lasers

Several pulsed lasers emitting in the near-infrared spectrum have been used for the treatment of leg veins, such as the alexandrite (755 nm), the diode (800 nm), and the Nd:YAG (1064 nm). Their longer wavelength provides deeper penetration into tissue, but their absorption by hemoglobin is less than with other vascular-specific lasers.

Intense pulsed light sources

The intense pulsed light sources (IPL) is a laser-like device that uses a flashlamp to produce a non-coherent pulsed light from 515 to 1200 nm at variable pulse durations and intervals. The use of filters in the hand piece eliminates various wavelengths and allows the physician to deliver a variety of wavelengths to better target vascular lesions. The major advantage of this device is its versatility given the wide range of wavelengths and pulse durations that allow treatment of deeper vascular lesions.[5]

Clinical applications

Despite the large variety of vascular-specific lasers, no single laser or light source can be used to treat all vascular lesions, and, in certain cases, more than one device is needed to treat a particular vascular disorder.

Port-wine stains

Significant clinical lightening of PWS can be achieved with the pulsed dye laser with only a few side effects.[6] The majority of patients require multiple treatment sessions to the same area to obtain maximal clearing. Approximately 75% of adult patients with PWS experience at least 50% lightening of lesions after a total of four treatments.[7] Pediatric PWS exhibit an even better response ranging from almost 100% clearing in all treated patients to at least 50% lightening in 87% of patients.[8] (261–264) More nodular or hypertrophic forms are best treated with the long-pulsed dye lasers or the quasi-continuous and continuous mode lasers. The rate of clearing of port-wine stains largely depends on their anatomic location, with lesions on the trunk and extremities responding less favorably compared with those on the head and neck. Also,

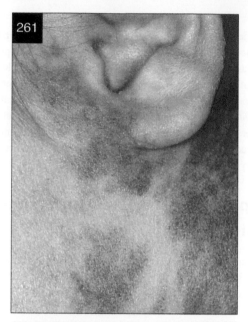

261: Childhood port-wine stain before treatment.
262: Childhood port-wine stain after a series of pulsed dye laser treatments.

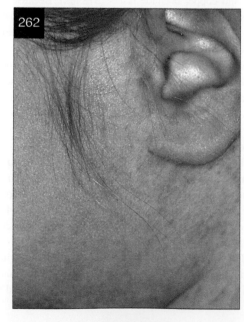

PWS located on the proximal extremities respond more rapidly than distal PWS, and midline PWS of the face clear faster than lesions located laterally. Furthermore, the more superficial red PWS respond better than the pink PWS in which the ectatic vessels are more deeply situated. In general, laser treatment of PWS should be initiated during infancy or early childhood in order to reduce the psychologic impact of the birthmark and to prevent hypertrophy as the lesion matures.

Hemangiomas

The pulsed dye laser is the treatment of choice for superficial hemangiomas, achieving maximal clearing after repetitive treatments.[9] Early initiation of treatment, either before or immediately after the onset of the proliferative stage, is

advocated to minimize rapid enlargement of the tumor, bleeding, ulceration, or obstruction of vital organs.[10] Thin lesions (≤3 mm thickness) usually respond with almost complete resolution, while lesions >3 mm are more resistant to treatment (**265, 266**). In ulcerated hemangiomas, which occur frequently in the perioral or perineal areas, pulsed dye laser therapy can promote healing and provide symptomatic relief.[11] Because of its limited skin penetration, the pulsed dye laser is not effective in treatment of the deep component of superficial

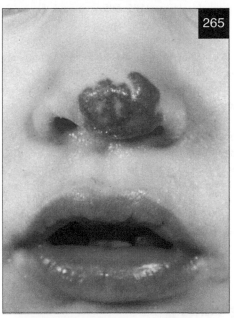

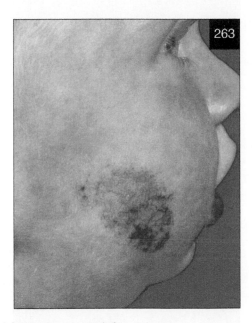

263: Infantile port-wine stain before treatment.
264: Infantile port-wine stain after a series of pulsed dye laser treatments.

265: Superficial hemangioma prior to treatment.
266: Superficial hemangioma after a series of pulsed dye laser treatments.

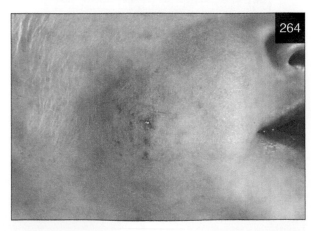

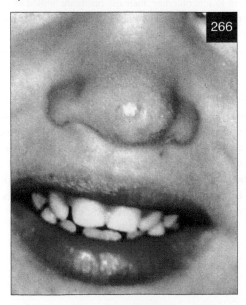

hemangiomas or of deep (cavernous) hemangiomas. These lesions are more likely to respond to treatment with the continuous-wave Nd:YAG laser, the newer long-pulsed dye lasers (595 nm, 1.5 ms), or the pulsed Nd:YAG lasers which have a more vascular selective tissue reaction.

Facial telangiectasia

Two approaches have been established for the treatment of telangiectasia with lasers, based on the existing laser devices: the pulsed dye lasers (585–595 nm), and the pulsed KTP lasers (532 nm). The original pulsed dye laser (585 nm, 450 μs) effectively treats facial telangiectasia as well as rosacea-associated telangiectasia and erythema, spider angiomas, telangiectasia associated with CREST syndrome, and generalized essential telangiectasia, but in every instance produces purpura. The newer long-pulsed duration pulse dye lasers are highly effective in the treatment of diffuse facial redness frequently seen in flushers and in individuals with rosacea, and in the treatment of facial telangiectasia (267, 268).[3] In both instances treatments can be performed with little or no purpura. The pulsed green light KTP lasers (532 nm) also clear facial telangiectasia by tracing them one by one. They do not produce purpura postoperatively, although the degree of clearing per treatment session is slightly less than with PDL.[12] Recently, the longer-wavelength infrared lasers, such as the Nd:YAG laser with a millisecond pulse duration, have been shown to be effective in treating facial telangiectasia.[13]

Leg veins

Until recently, lasers and light sources were used as an adjuvant treatment to sclerotherapy, their use primarily limited to vessels <1.2 mm in diameter. The pulsed KTP lasers (532 nm), the pulsed dye lasers (585–595 nm) and the pulsed light source (515–1200 nm) have been employed for the treatment of leg veins, but their use has been hampered by incomplete vessel clearance and a high incidence of post-treatment pigmentary alterations (269–272).[14] Recent studies, using near-infrared lasers (alexandrite laser, 755 nm, 3 ms; diode laser, 810 nm, 30–40 ms; long-pulsed Nd:YAG laser, 1064 nm, 10–16 ms) with deeper penetrating wavelengths and higher fluences in conjunction with various epidermal cooling methods have demonstrated good responses in larger diameter (up to 2–3 mm) and more deeply situated leg telangiectasia and reticular veins.[13, 16, 17] Sclerotherapy remains the treatment of choice for most leg veins.

Other vascular lesions

A great variety of vascular lesions have been treated effectively with the available laser devices, such as pyogenic granulomas, poikiloderma of Civatte, venous lakes, cherry angiomas, and spider angiomas.[18]

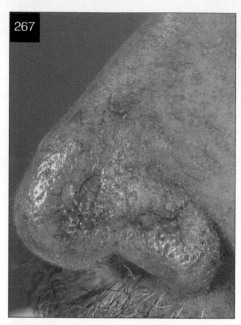

267: Diffuse erythema with telangiectasia prior to treatment.
268: This individual could have been treated with equal success with the pulsed dye laser with or without purpura, with an intense pulselight source, or with a pulsed 532 nm source.

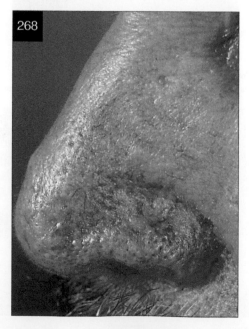

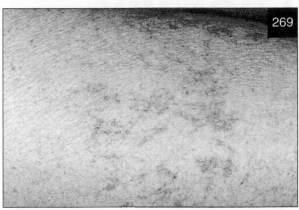

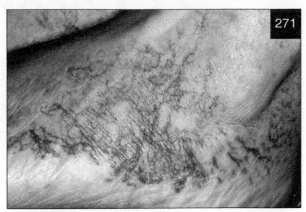

269, 270: Fine telangiectasia of the thigh (269) fine telangiectasia of the thigh after two treatments with a long-pulsed 1064 nm laser (270).

271, 272: Fine ectatic veins over the lateral aspect of the foot prior to treatment (271) after a series of treatments usine a continuous wave dye laser using the tracing technique (272).

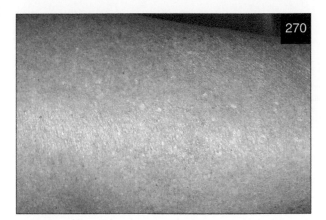

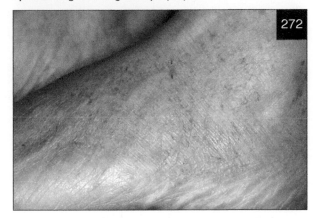

References

1. Anderson RR, Parrish JA. Selective photothermolysis: precise microsurgery by selective absorption of pulsed radiation. *Science* 1983;**220**:524–7.

2. Tan OT, Morrison P, Kurban AK. 585 nm for the treatment of port-wine stains. *Plast Reconstr Surg* 1990;**86**;1112–17.

3. Alam M, Dover JS, Arndt KA. Treatment of facial telangiectasia with variable pulse high-fluence pulsed dye laser: comparison of efficacy with fluences immediately below and above the purpura threshold. *Dermatol Surg* 2003;**29**:681-5.

4. Clark C, Cameron H, Moseley H, Ferguson J, Ibbotson SH. Treatment of superficial cutaneous vascular lesions: experience with the KTP 532 nm laser. *Lasers Med Sci* 2004;**19**:1-5.

5. Angermeier MC. Treatment of facial vascular lesions with intense pulsed light source. *J Cutan Laser Ther* 1999;**1**:95–100.

6. Scherer K, Lorenz S, Wimmershoff M, Landthaler M, Hohenleutner U. Both the flashlamp-pumped dye laser and the long-pulsed tunable dye laser can improve results in port-wine stain therapy. *Br J Dermatol* 2001;**145**:79–84.

7. Garden JM, Polla LL, Tan OT. The treatment of portwine stains by the pulsed dye laser: analysis of pulse duration and long-term therapy. *Arch Dermatol* 1988;**124**:889–96.

8. Reyes BA, Geronemus RG. Treatment of port wine stains with the flashlamp-pumped pulse dye laser. *J Am Acad Dermatol* 1990;**23**;1142–8.

9. Poetke M, Philipp C, Berlien HP. Flashlamp-pumped pulsed dye laser for hemangiomas in infancy: treatment of superficial vs mixed hemangiomas. *Arch Dermatol* 2000;**136**:628–32.

10. Al Buainian, Verhaeghe E, Dierckxsens L, Naeyaert JM. Early treatment of hemangiomas with lasers. A review. *Dermatology* 2003;**206**:370-373.

11. David LR, Malek MM, Argenta LC. Efficacy of pulse dye laser therapy for the treatment of ulcerated haemangiomas: a review of 78 patients. *Br J Plast Surg* 2003;**56**:317–27.

12. Kauvar AN, Frew KE, Friedman PM, Geronemus RG. Cooling gel improves KTP laser treatment of facial telangiectasia. *Lasers Surg Med* 2002;**30**:149–53.

13. Sarradet DM, Hussain M, Goldberg DJ. Millisecond 1064-nm neodymium: YAG laser treatment of facial telangiectasia. *Dermatol Surg* 2003;**29**:56–8.

14. Kauvar ANB. The role of lasers in the treatment of leg veins. *Semin Cutan Med Surg* 2000;**19**:245–52.

15. Brunnberg S, Lorenz S, Landthaler M, Hohenleutner U. Evaluation of the long-pulsed high fluence alexandrite laser therapy of leg telangiectasia. *Lasers Surg Med* 2002;**31**:359–62.

16. Sadick NS, Prieto VG, Shea CR, Nicholson J, McCaffrey T. Clinical and pathophysiologic correlates of 1064-nm Nd:Yag laser treatment of reticular veins and venulectasias. *Arch Dermatol* 2001;**137**:613–17.

17. Omura NE, Dover JS, Arndt KA, Kauvar AN. Treatment of reticular veins with a 1064 nm long-pulsed Nd:YAG laser. *J Am Acad Dermatol* 2003;**48**:76–81.

18. Rothfleisch JE, Kosann MK, Levine VJ, Ashinoff R. Laser treatment of congenital and acquired vascular lesions. A review. *Dermatol Clin* 2002;**20**:1–18.

23 Laser Therapy for Pigmented Lesions and Tattoos

Alexander J Stratigos and Jeffrey S Dover

The approach to the treatment of pigmented lesions with lasers depends on the anatomic location of pigment (epidermal, dermal or mixed), the nature of pigment (endogenous or exogenous), and its tissue distribution (extracellular, intracellular). In most pigmented lesions, the chromophore is melanin, although other exogenous and endogenous pigments can be targeted. In order to achieve specificity, it is necessary to use wavelengths that avoid absorption by other skin chromophores and penetrate to the desired depth. A selective window for targeting melanin lies between 630 nm and 1100 nm, where there is good skin penetration and preferential absorption of melanin over oxyhemoglobin. Short wavelengths (<600 nm) can damage only superficial pigmented lesions leaving deeper structures intact, while longer wavelengths (>600 nm) can target pigmented lesions in the dermis, such as nevi of Ota, and most tattoos. Pigment specificity of lasers is not only wavelength dependent, but also pulse width dependent. The determination of the appropriate pulse duration is primarily based on the size of the target and its thermal relaxation time. The primary site of laser-induced damage is most likely the melanosome, the intracellular organelle in which melanin is synthesized and stored.[1] With an estimated thermal relaxation time that ranges from 250 to 1000 ns, depending on their size, melanosomes require nanosecond laser pulses (<1 μs) for their selective disruption. Recent evidence, however, suggests that longer pulse durations, in the millisecond range, may effectively remove epidermal pigmentation, especially in individuals with darker skin complexion.[2]

Types of lasers and light sources

The lasers we currently use to treat pigmented lesions are grouped into four categories: the highly selective or Q-switched (QS) lasers and some longer pulsed lasers, the less pigment-selective lasers (continuous and quasi-continuous wave lasers), the non-pigment specific or resurfacing lasers (CO_2 and erbium:YAG lasers), and the intense pulsed light source. The Q-switched lasers include the Q-switched ruby laser at 694 nm (pulse duration of 25–40 ns), the Q-switched alexandrite at 755 nm (50–100 ns), and the Q-switched Nd:YAG laser at 1064 nm (5–7 ns), all of which can target epidermal and deeper dermal pigment. In addition, the Q-switched frequency doubled Nd:YAG at 532 nm (pulse duration of 5–7 ns) and longer pulsed millisecond domain 532 nm lasers emit shorter wavelengths that target epidermal pigment abnormalities.

Mechanism of action of Q-switched lasers

Q-switched lasers emit high-powered pulses with extremely short pulse durations – in the nanosecond range – that selectively target exogenous or endogenous pigment with minimal collateral damage to the neighboring tissue. The primary subcellular event after irradiation with a Q-switched laser is the thermomechanical destruction of melanosomes, which is followed by the production of acoustic waves and the eventual destruction of pigmented keratinocytes or melanocytes.

Clinical applications

In general, laser-treated lentigines, ephelids and dermal melanocytoses improve markedly or clear completely, while café-au-lait macules, postinflammatory hyperpigmentation, and melasma exhibit variable responses to laser treatment.[3]

Epidermal pigmented lesions (Table 23.1)
Superficial pigmented lesions, such as ephelids, solar and labial lentigines (**273, 274**) and flat-pigmented seborrheic keratoses, can be effectively treated with any of the Q-switched lasers. One or two treatment sessions are usually sufficient to clear

most lentigines, although further treatments are occasionally required for more resistant lesions. The absence of purpura following treatment with the Q-switched ruby (694 nm) and alexandrite (755 nm) lasers makes them slightly preferable over the shorter wavelength or green light lasers, particularly in the case of facial lesions. Postoperative pigmentary changes, such as hyperpigmentation and hypopigmentation, are not uncommon particularly in skin type III and IV individuals, as well as in sun-tanned individuals.

Café-au-lait macules

The response of café-au-lait macules (CALM) to Q-switched laser therapy is variable and often unpredictable. Short-term lightening or complete clearing is frequently seen after repeated Q-switched laser treatments but, despite initial improvement, recurrences are frequent, occurring in as many as 50% of cases (**275, 276**).

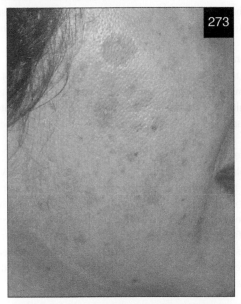

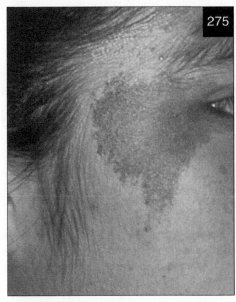

273, 274: Lentigenes on the cheeks prior to treatment (273) after a single treatment with the Q-switched ruby laser (274). The patient was satisfied with the degree of improvement achieved, although further treatment would have produced even further, if not complete, lightening.

275, 276: Café-au-lait macule of the cheek prior to treatment (275); after a series of Q-switched laser treatments (276) (courtesy of Dr Tezuka Tedashi).

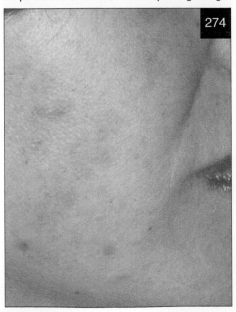

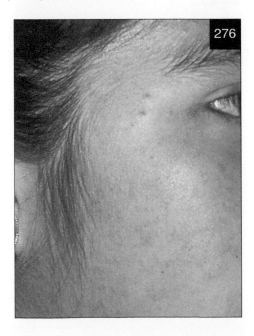

Melasma

Despite repeated attempts using Q-switched lasers in the treatment of melasma, longstanding clearing has rarely been achieved and recurrence is the rule in almost all cases. The epidermal type of melasma shows a modest response to laser treatment similar to that seen with bleaching preparations and chemical peels. The dermal and mixed types of melasma are generally non-responsive to laser therapy. Successful results in clearing dermal-type melasma have been reported, however with a combination of pulsed CO_2 laser resurfacing followed by Q-switched alexandrite laser treatment to selectively remove the dermal melanin.

Nevus of Ota/Ito

Q-switched laser therapy has now become the treatment of choice for dermal pigmented lesions, such as the nevus of Ota, the nevus of Ito, and the Mongolian spot (277, 278).[4,5] The Q-switched ruby laser, the Q-switched alexandrite laser, and the Q-switched Nd:YAG laser at 1064 nm are all highly effective in targeting the deep dermal melanocytes and, in the case of nevus of Ota, produce significant (>75%) or complete lesion clearing after an average of 4–8 laser treatments with fluences ranging from 5–12 J/cm^2.[6] With the exception of temporal postinflammatory hyperpigmentation, no serious side effects have been reported after laser treatment, and once the nevus has fully resolved, recurrences are rare.

Drug-induced hyperpigmentation

Drug-induced hyperpigmentation may also improve with the use of short-pulsed lasers. A typical example is the blue-black hyperpigmentation caused by minocycline, which has been shown to dramatically clear by virtually all Q-switched lasers (ruby, alexandrite, and Nd:YAG at 1064 nm).[7] A similar result has been reported with amiodarone-induced hyperpigmentation treated with the Q-switched ruby laser.[8] In these cases, laser treatment should be deferred until the offending agent has been discontinued and sufficient time has elapsed to allow for spontaneous resolution of most of the pigmentation.

Postinflammatory hyperpigmentation

Laser treatment of postinflammatory hyperpigmentation has been unsatisfactory. Although some degree of lightening may be seen initially, recurrences or even worsening of the pigmentation from the added laser injury may occur in susceptible individuals.

Becker's nevi

Variable results have been observed in Becker's nevi, in which hyperpigmentation and hypertrichosis are the principal patient concerns. Despite multiple Q-switched laser treatments, pigmentary changes, incomplete removal and recurrence occur frequently. At present the preferred treatment approach for these lesions is the combination of a Q-switched laser and a longer pulsed, pigment-specific laser to remove both the macular pigmentation and the hair of Becker's nevi.

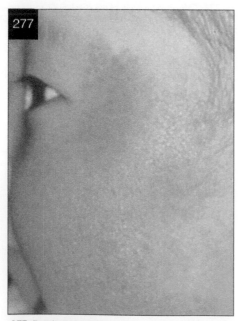

277: Facial nevus of Ota prior to treatment

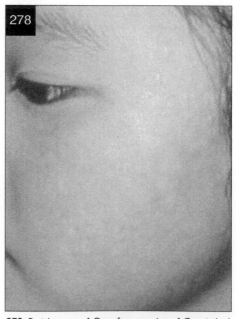

278: Facial nevus of Ota after a series of Q-switched laser treatments (courtesy of Dr Tezuka Tedashi).

Nevi spili

Nevi spili have an inconsistent response to laser treatment, with their deeply pigmented portion (junctional or nevus portion) responding better than their macular portion (epidermal or café-au-lait portion). Complete or near-complete clearing (>80%) has been reported after an average of three to four treatment sessions using a Q-switched ruby laser treatment (694 nm, 5.5–10 J/cm²),[9] although other reports show a less favorable outcome with incomplete clearing and frequent recurrences, particularly of the macular portion of the lesion.

Congenital and acquired nevomelanocytic nevi

Studies assessing the efficacy of the Q-switched ruby in small- to medium-sized congenital nevi have shown partial clinical improvement after several sessions and frequent recurrences.[10] These results could be interpreted by the histologic examination of laser-treated lesions where, despite the overall reduction in nevi cells, residual nevomelanocytes remained unaffected in the deeper dermis. Long-pulse, pigment-specific lasers have also been used in the treatment of melanocytic nevi. In one study of eight Japanese patients with congenital nevi who were treated with a long-pulsed ruby laser with or without a Q-switched ruby laser, eight of ten lesions showed significant lightening of their pigmentation despite the histologic presence of residual nevi cells in the deeper dermis.[11] No evidence of malignant degeneration was observed in the treated areas up to 8 years after laser treatment. Due to the lack of studies with long-term follow-up, the role of lasers in the treatment of nevomelanocytic lesions remains to be elucidated.

Tattoos (Table 23.2)

The absorption of laser energy by the tattoo possibly causes fragmentation of the ink particles, which are then eliminated either externally through scale or crust or systemically through the lymphatic drainage or rephagocytosis by tissue macrophages.[12] Treatment of tattoos with lasers depends on the type of tattoo and its pigment content. There is no single laser that can treat all colors and hence, multicolored tattoos usually require the use of more than one laser for complete removal. Black tattoo pigment absorbs all laser wavelengths, while green tattoo pigment is best treated with the Q-switched ruby (694 nm) and alexandrite (755 nm) lasers. Red tattoo pigment is more effectively treated with the pigmented dye laser (510 nm) and the frequency doubled Q-switched Nd:YAG (532 nm). Amateur tattoos require fewer laser treatments than professional tattoos that are more densely pigmented and usually contain multiple pigments (**279, 280**). Anatomic location and age of tattoo may also influence the response to laser therapy. Tattoos located on the distal extremities usually require more treatments than proximally located tattoos, possibly due to decreased lymphatic drainage in the periphery. In addition, older tattoos may be easier to remove than fresh tattoos because they contain less dense pigment deposits.[13] Traumatic tattoos typically respond well to Q-switched lasers because of their predominantly superficial location and carbon-based pigment.[14] Longer treatment intervals (≥2 months) are currently recommended for maximal removal of the tattoo particles by macrophages.

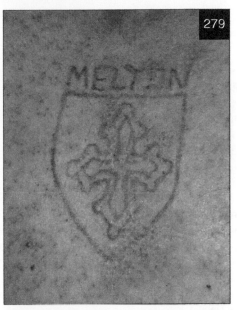

279: Amateur tattoo prior to treatment.
280: Amateur tattoo after four Q-switched Nd:YAG laser treatments.

Table 23.1: **Q-switched lasers for pigmented lesions**

Laser type	Wavelength (nm)	Pulse width (ns)
Q-switched ruby laser	694	25
Q-switched alexandrite	755	50–100
Q-switched Nd:YAG	1064	5–15
	532	5–15

Table 23.2: **Q-switched lasers for different colors of tattoo ink**

Tattoo ink colour	Laser
Blue/black	QS-ruby (694 nm), QS-alexandrite (755 nm), QS-Nd:YAG (1064 nm)
Green	QS-alexandrite (755 nm), QS-ruby (694 nm)
Red/orange/purple	QS-frequency doubled Nd:YAG (532 nm), pigmented pulsed dye (510 nm)
Yellow	Pigmented pulsed dye (510 nm)

References

1. Polla LL, Margolis RJ, Dover JS et al. Melanosomes are a primary target of Q-switched ruby laser irradiation in guinea pig skin. *J Invest Dermatol* 1987;**89**:281–6.

2. Rosenbach A, Lee SR, John RH. Treatment of medium-brown solar lentigines using an alexandrite laser designed for hair reduction. *Arch Dermatol* 2002;**138**:547–8.

3. Stratigos AJ, Dover JS, Arndt KA. Laser treatment of pigmented lesions-2000. How far have we gone? *Arch Dermatol* 2000;**136**:915–21.

4. Watanabe S, Takahashi H. Treatment of Nevus of Ota with the Q-switched ruby laser. *N Engl J Med* 1994;**331**:1745–50.

5. Kono T, Chan HH, Ercocen AR et al. Use of Q-switched ruby laser in the treatment of nevus of ota in different age groups. *Lasers Surg Med* 2003;**32**:391–5.

6. Alster TS, Williams CM. Treatment of nevus of Ota by the Q-switched alexandrite laser. *Dermatol Surg* 1995;**21**:592–6.

7. Green D, Friedman KJ. Treatment of minocycline-induced cutaneous pigmentation with the Q-switched Alexandrite laser and a review of the literature. *J Am Acad Dermatol* 2001;**44**:342–7.

8. Karrer S, Hohenleutner U, Szeimies RM, Landthaler M. Amiodarone-induced pigmentation resolves after treatment with the Q-switched ruby laser. *Arch Dermatol* 1999;**135**:251–3.

9. Grevelink JM, Gonzalez S, Bonoan R, Vibhagool C, Gonzalez E. Treatment of nevus spilus with the Q-switched ruby laser. *Dermatol Surg* 1997;**23**:365–9.

10. Waldorf HA, Kauvar AN, Geronemus RG. Treatment of small and medium congenital nevi with the Q-switched ruby laser. *Arch Dermatol* 1996;**132**:301–4.

11. Imayama S, Ueda S. Long- and short-term histological observations of congenital nevi treated with the normal-mode ruby laser. *Arch Dermatol* 1999;**135**:1211–18.

12. Kuperman-Beade M, Levine VJ, Ashinoff R. Laser removal of tattoos. *Am J Clin Dermatol* 2001;**2**:21–5.

13. Kilmer SL. Laser eradication of pigmented lesions and tattoos. *Clin Dermatol* 2002;**20**:37–53.

14. Prinz BM, Vavricka SR, Graf P, Burg G, Dummer R. Efficacy of laser treatment of tattoos using lasers emitting wavelenghts of 532 nm, 755 nm, and 1064 nm. *Br J Dermatol* 2004;**150**:245-251.

24
Ablative and Non-ablative Laser Skin Resurfacing

Alexander J Stratigos and Jeffrey S Dover

Over the past decade, laser skin resurfacing (LSR) has dramatically altered our approach to facial rejuvenation. The development of ablative resurfacing with the CO_2 and the erbium:YAG lasers has greatly enhanced our ability to treat photodamaged skin layer by layer by precisely removing it layer by layer in a precisely controlled manner, while leaving behind a very narrow zone of thermal damage. Non-ablative laser and light treatments provide an alternative to the traditional ablative modalities and improve the overall skin texture and tone with limited downtime after each treatment.

Ablative laser skin resurfacing

Ablative resurfacing improves skin roughness, fine and moderately deep facial wrinkles, and dyspigmentation by replacing the epidermis and superficial dermis with a new papillary dermis and overlying epidermis.

Types of lasers
The two main resurfacing lasers are the carbon dioxide laser and the erbium:YAG laser.

Carbon dioxide (CO_2) laser
The CO_2 laser emits at 10,600 nm, a wavelength that is strongly absorbed by tissue water (absorption coefficient of 800/cm²). With a pulse duration of <1 ms, CO_2 laser light penetrates only 30 μm into tissue, and leaves a thin layer of residual thermal damage of 100–150 μm of tissue.[1] By using these parameters, the CO_2 lasers can precisely control the depth of ablation and thermal damage by combining high peak powers with short pulses. Two basic CO_2 laser systems have been used in cutaneous resurfacing: the high-powered pulsed CO_2 laser, which delivers its energy in the form of individual pulses of 600 μs–1 ms duration, and the scanned CO_2 lasers, which use a

rapidly scanning focused beam. Despite their technical differences, both laser systems achieve equivalent clinical results.

Erbium:YAG (Er:YAG) laser
The normal mode Er:YAG laser emits pulses of infrared light at 2940 nm, a wavelength close to the absorption peak of water. This results in an absorption coefficient that is 16 times that of the CO_2 laser and in a much shallower tissue penetration (about 1 μm of tissue versus 20 μm penetration depth of the CO_2 laser). The combination of these two factors results in a more precise ablation of skin with minimal thermal damage to the surrounding tissues (estimated residual thermal damage zone of 10–40 μm). Er:YAG laser resurfacing has been associated with decreased discomfort during the procedure and faster healing times postoperatively compared to the CO_2 laser systems. However, it does not appear to produce the same amount of tissue tightening or contraction, which influences its ability for long-term improvement of photo-aged skin.[2] The variable pulse Er:YAG laser with pulse widths of 10–50 μm has been recently introduced in clinical practices demonstrating immediate tissue contraction and a healing rate that is intermediate between that of the short-pulsed Er:YAG and the resurfacing CO_2 lasers. Clinical studies comparing the variable pulse Er:YAG laser with the CO_2 have shown that the degree of wrinkle improvement was similar, although slightly superior with the CO_2 laser[3]

Clinical indications
The two most popular indications of laser skin resurfacing are photo-aging and acne scarring. Photo-aging and its associated skin changes, for example rhytides, dyschromias, solar lentigines, and actinic keratoses, respond very favorably to LSR. The improvement is usually more marked for fine and superficial rhytides, particularly those on the perioral and periorbital areas, and less pronounced for deeper wrinkles

and dynamic creases (**281, 282**). Laser resurfacing is also effective for elevated or depressed distensible acne scars in which the fibrotic tissue can be removed or the edges of the scars can be "sculpted" by ablation (**283, 284**). At the same time tightening of the skin enhances the appearance of atrophic acne scars. Ice-picked or bound-down scars respond less favorably.⁴ Crateriform varicella scars and other skin disorders can also be improved with laser resurfacing *(Table 24.1)*.

Patient selection

The ideal laser resurfacing candidate is a healthy, fair-skinned patient with realistic expectations. Potential contraindications include keloid formation and conditions that reduce the num-

ber of adnexal structures, for example prior radiation therapy or scleroderma. Prior isotretinoin therapy has been associated with atypical scar formation after dermabrasion and, therefore, it is recommended that patients postpone laser resurfacing for at least 1 year after isotretinoin discontinuation.

Preoperative course

Daily use of topical tretinoin or an alfa-hydroxy-acid preparation for 4–6 weeks prior to resurfacing has been advocated to speed re-epithelialization. Antiviral prophylaxis is instituted in all patients undergoing the procedure, regardless of whether they report a history of herpes labialis. Perioperative oral antibiotics with Gram-positive coverage are also prescribed to reduce the risk of bacterial infection.

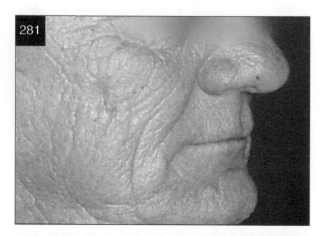

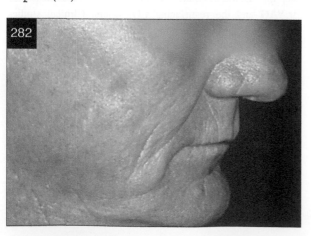

281, 282: A 50-year-old man with severe photo-aging prior to laser skin resurfacing (281) 6 months after laser skin resurfacing with the UltraPulse CO_2 laser (282).

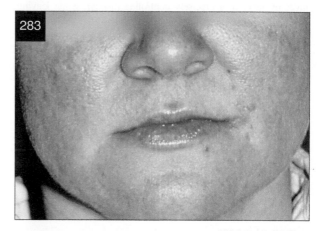

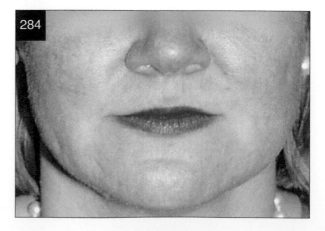

283, 284: A woman in her late 20s with atrophic acne scars prior to laser skin resurfacing (283) 1 year after laser skin resurfacing with the UltraPulse CO_2 laser (284).

Anesthesia

For patients who undergo treatment of one or two cosmetic units, such as the perioral or periorbital areas, local anesthesia is sufficient. For full face laser CO_2 resurfacing, a combination regimen of intramuscular or intravenous sedation in addition to nerve blocks plus topical or injectable anesthetics is commonly used. Topical anesthetic products can be used as supplemental agents to local or regional anesthesia for superficial laser procedures, particularly with the Er:YAG laser.

Technique

In CO_2 laser resurfacing for wrinkles, successive "passes" of single vaporizing laser pulses with minimal overlap are performed with gentle but thorough wiping of the desiccated proteinaceous debris in between laser passes. In a normal resurfacing session, two passes are made with the CO_2 laser over the entire treated area. Subsequent passes are concentrated on high points of scars or shoulders of rhytides. The endpoint of treatment is the effacement of tissue irregularities and visible wrinkles. In resurfacing with the traditional Er:YAG laser, several passes (up to four) are required to remove the epidermal layer, and as many as eight to ten passes are needed to reach the desired endpoint, namely the effacement of rhytides or pinpoint bleeding. Wiping of the desiccated proteinaceous material is not generally needed, except perhaps after the first pass. Visible wound contraction seldom occurs in resurfacing with the traditional Er:YAG laser, but does occur with the variable pulse Er:YAG laser (10–50 ms).

Table 24.1: Indications for laser resurfacing CO_2 and erbium:YAG lasers

Benign skin lesions	Premalignant skin lesions
• Rhytides, facial	• Actinic cheilitis
• Rhytides, non-facial (Er:YAG only)	• Actinic keratoses
• Epidermal nevi	• Bowen's disease
• Rhinophyma	• Erythroplasia of Queyrat
• Atrophic acne scars	• Superficial basal cell carcinoma
• Varicella scars	
• Solar lentigines, facial	
• Syringomas	
• Tricho-epitheliomas	
• Xanthelasma	
• Hypertrophic scars	
• Adenoma sebaceum	
• Sebaceous hyperplasia	
• Seborrheic keratosis	

Postoperative course

During the first few days after laser resurfacing there is a significant amount of exudates and edema. Patients are encouraged to apply frequently compresses with 0.25% acetic acid, normal saline, or cool tap water soaks followed by the application of a healing ointment to the treated areas. The use of bio-occlusive dressings during the first 24–72 hours has been shown to promote re-epithelialization and alleviate patient discomfort. Antibiotic coverage against Gram-positive bacteria is continued for a minimum of 5 days postoperatively and oral antiviral prophylaxis is continued until re-epithelialization is complete (10–14 days). Following re-epithelialization, there is a variable period of erythema that ranges from 1 to 4 months. Sun avoidance is essential during the entire period of post-laser erythema to reduce the risk of postinflammatory hyperpigmentation.

Side effects and complications

Side effects following CO_2 laser resurfacing are frequent and predictable. They can be divided into six categories: immediate/predictable effects, infectious, dermatitic, follicular, pigmentary, and scarring changes (Table 24.2).

Non-ablative laser and light therapy

Non-ablative laser and light therapy (also termed photorejuvenation, PhotoFacial, laser toning, subsurface resurfacing) is a relatively new concept for the improvement of the visual appearance of photodamaged and acne-scarred skin. The entire concept is based on early studies that found that the pulsed dye laser induced a Grenz zone of new healthy-appearing collagen deposited in the papillary dermis after just

Table 24.2: Q-switched lasers for pigmented lesions

Side effects	Symptoms and signs
Predictable	Oozing, crusting, edema, erythema, pruritus, skin tightness
Infectious	Bacterial, viral, yeast infection
Dermatitis	Eczematous, allergic contact
Follicular	Acne, acneiform eruption, milia, perioral dermatitis
Pigmentary	Hyperpigmentation, permanent delayed hypopigmentation
Scarring	Atrophic, hypertrophic , keloidal

one treatment with relatively low energy settings. A number of different wavelengths and devices have been found to effectively enhance the appearance of aged skin. Among the conditions that can be addressed are erythema and telangiectasia, pigmentation, lentigines, and textural imperfection from fine to moderate rhytides to other surface irregularities such as acne scarring. A major attraction of non-ablative therapy is the very limited downtime after each treatment.

Non-ablative laser devices

Numerous laser and light devices,[5] including the KTP laser (532 nm), pulsed dye laser (585 nm, 595 nm), intense pulsed light (IPL) devices (515–1200 nm), Nd:YAG lasers (1064 nm Q-switched, 1064 nm long-pulse, 1319 nm, 1320 nm), diode lasers (980 nm, 1450 nm), Er:Glass laser (1540 nm), and light-emitting diodes, have been adapted to be effective in, or specifically developed for, non-ablative resurfacing (Table 24.3). The mid-infrared devices, including 1320, 1450, and 1540 nm devices, appear most effective for wrinkle and acne scar reduction. Red color and vascular lesions are best addressed by vascular-selective devices, such as the KTP, pulsed-dye, and long-pulsed Nd:YAG lasers. The KTP also has efficacy for pigmentation as does the Q-switched Nd:YAG laser, but IPL devices, by virtue of their broad emission spectrum, appear the most effective for simultaneous treatment of both red and brown patches.

Tissue effects of non-ablative therapy

For non-ablative therapy, an epidermal surface temperature of 40–48°C is ideal since this correlates with a dermal temperature of 55–65°C, which is required for collagen denaturation. In histologic analyses of treated skin, dermal thickening is observed which is interpreted as "increased" and "organized" horizontally arrayed bundles of normal collagen fibers in the papillary dermis. This finding may result from trauma and inflammation caused during remodeling after thermal or light injury to the dermis.[6,7] Whether the alterations produced by non-ablative laser are as persistent as typical photodamage, and the extent to which they are comparable to photodamage, is not known.[8]

Clinical efficacy

Clinical evaluations of non-ablative laser therapy are mainly performed through patient and physician evaluations, photographic evaluations and objective non-invasive texture measurement methods (profilometry, ultrasound, three-dimensional in vivo skin imaging systems).[3] Although differences between "before and after" results can be subtle and not always seen easily, the popularity of this treatment among patients and physicians strongly suggests that these differences are likely to be real. Cumulative aesthetic benefits from non-ablative resurfacing are similar in type though less in magnitude than the results of ablative resurfacing.

Table 24.3: Non-ablative lasers and light sources for skin rejuvenation

Laser type	Wavelength (nm)	Indications (other than skin tone improvement)
KTP	532	Erythema, telangiectasia, vascular lesions
Pulsed dye	585, 595	Erythema, telangiectasia, vascular lesions
Q-switched Nd:YAG	1064	Pigmentary disorders
Long-pulsed Nd:YAG	1064 1319 1320	Erythema, telangiectasia, vascular lesions Wrinkles, acne scars, surface irregularities Wrinkles, acne scars, surface irregularities
Diode	980 1450	Erythema, telangiectasia, vascular lesions Wrinkles, acne scars, surface irregularities
Er:Glass	1540	Wrinkles, acne scars, surface irregularities
Intense pulsed light (IPL)	515–1200	Vascular and pigmented lesions

Patient selection

Good candidates for non-ablative resurfacing tend to be relatively young, usually 25–65 years of age, and have minimal sagging of the face.[9] It is essential for patients to understand that skin texture will improve and fine lines in particular will be softened, not eradicated. Additionally, since changes will occur gradually, typically after three to six or more treatments, those receiving non-ablative treatments should not expect dramatic results immediately. Patients who wish to minimize treatment discomfort and downtime, or those who wish to be on a maintenance therapy for the texture and color of their facial skin, tend to be more satisfied with non-ablative resurfacing. Dark-skinned patients or those with a tendency to develop hyperpigmentation after skin injury can often safely undergo non-ablative infrared therapy, although the risk of pigmentary changes in such patients is still greater than in lighter-skinned patients.

Perioperative considerations

Treatment with non-ablative lasers is variably painful. The infrared sources are the most painful and usually require topical anesthesia for the procedures to be tolerable.

Mild erythema and edema do occur following each treatment, and vary in intensity and duration depending on the device used. Infrared lasers (1320 nm, 1450 nm, 1540 nm), while uncomfortable, are associated with only a few hours of redness and swelling, while side effects and longer duration tissue effects are routine with the other devices, such as the pulsed dye lasers, IPL sources, and 532 and 1064 nm Nd:YAG lasers.

Future directions for non-ablative therapy

As the mechanisms underlying non-ablative therapy are better understood, these treatments may be adapted to exploit these biochemical and physical changes.[10]

Also, combined rejuvenation regimens that incorporate non-ablative resurfacing will likely be further perfected. Botulinum toxin, soft tissue augmentation materials, glycolic acid peels, and other abrasion techniques can be combined with non-ablative resurfacing in order to achieve a rosier glow of the skin and a smoother skin texture.

References

1. Walsh JT, Flotte TJ, Anderson RR, Deutsch TF. Pulsed CO_2 laser tissue ablation: effect of tissue type and pulse duration on thermal damage. *Lasers Surg Med* 1988;**8**:108–18.

2. Ross VE, McKinlay JR, Anderson RR. Why does carbon dioxide resurfacing work? *Arch Dermatol* 1999;**135**:444–54.

3. Newman JB, Lord JL, Ash K, McDaniel DH. Variable pulse erbium:YAG laser skin resurfacing of perioral rhytides and side-by-side comparison with carbon dioxide laser. *Lasers Surg Med* 2000;**26**:208–14.

4. Jacob CI, Dover JS, Kaminer MS. Acne scarring: a classification system and review of treatment options. *J Am Acad Dermatol* 2001;**45**:109–17.

5. Kelly, Kristen M, Majaron B, Nelson S. Nonablative laser and light rejuvenation. The newest approach to photodamaged skin. *Arch Facial Plast Surg* 2001;**3**:230-235.

6. Alam M, Hsu TS, Dover JS, Wrone DA, Arndt KA. Non-ablative laser and light treatments: histology and tissue effects–a review. *Lasers Surg Med* 2003;**33**:30-9.

7. Schmults CD, Phelps R, Goldberg DJ. Nonablative facial remodeling: erythema reduction and histologic evidence of new collagen formation using a 300-microsecond 1064-nm Nd:YAG laser. *Arch Dermatol* 2004;**140**:1373-1376.

8. Kopera D, Smolle J, Kaddu S, Kerl H. Nonablative laser treatment of wrinkles: meeting the objective? Assessment by 25 dermatologists. *Br J Dermatol* 2004;**150**:936-939.

9. Alam M, Dover JS. Non-ablative laser and light therapy: an approach to patient and device selection. *Skin Therapy Lett* 2003;**8**:4–7.

10. Alam M, Hsu TS, Dover JS, Wrone DA, Arndt KA. Energy delivery devices for cutaneous remodeling: lasers, lights, and radio waves. *Arch Dermatol* 2003;**139**:1351–60.

25 Laser Hair Removal

Alexander J Stratigos, Jeffrey S Dover and Harry Moseley

Laser hair removal has now become one of the most frequently performed laser procedures, providing safe and effective hair removal from large body surfaces. In contrast to conventional methods, laser hair removal induces long-lasting hair growth delay and is associated with low treatment discomfort.

Modes of laser-induced hair damage

In order to achieve hair growth arrest and permanent inhibition of new hair formation, both regenerating centers of the hair follicle, the "bulge" and the hair bulb, must be destroyed by the laser. There are three means by which light can cause follicular damage: photothermal, photomechanical (through exogenous pigment particles) or photochemical (topical photodynamic therapy). Photothermal injury is the principal mechanism of action for most currently available lasers. It thermally destroys the follicle by targeting the principal follicular melanin, which is extensively distributed in the hair shaft, the follicular epithelium, and the heavily melanized matrix cells. Lasers causing photothermal hair destruction usually emit in the red to infrared spectrum (600–1100 nm) because at these wavelengths they combine selective absorption by melanin and deep penetration in the dermis. To achieve spatial confinement of thermal damage, their pulse duration is equal to or less than the thermal relaxation time of the hair follicle (estimated to be 10–100 ms, depending on size). The use of lasers for hair removal has been combined with selective cooling of the epidermis by a large variety of means in an effort to reduce epidermal injury from concomitant absorption by epidermal melanin.[1]

Types of lasers

Laser hair removal systems are typically grouped in three categories, depending on their wavelength and type of light sources: red light lasers (ruby laser, 694 nm), infrared light lasers (alexandrite, 755 nm; diode, 800 nm; Nd:YAG, 1064 nm),[2-4] and intense pulsed light sources (515–1200 nm).[5] Since these lasers or light sources target follicular melanin, they are most effective and safe for fair-skinned individuals with dark-colored hair.

Clinical responses

Two follicular responses are seen after laser treatment: temporary hair growth arrest and long-standing hair removal.[6] Temporary hair growth arrest lasting for 1–3 months occurs in all patients regardless of hair color (with the exception perhaps of white hair). Long-standing or permanent hair removal is mainly dependent on hair color and fluences used (Table 25.1). The ideal treatment parameters vary among the different laser devices, although most of them need a critical fluence threshold for permanent hair reduction.[7] The majority of patients with brown or black coarse terminal hair treated with high fluences (>30 J/cm^2) and large spot sizes using the ruby, alexandrite or diode laser will have permanent hair reduction with an average of 15–35% long-term hair loss after each laser treatment (285, 286).[8] Regrowing hair is often reduced in number and has a thinner and lighter appearance than the original hair, which contributes to the overall improvement. Other follicular disorders, for example pseudofolliculitis barbae and acne, have also been shown to benefit from laser hair removal.[9]

Treatment considerations

Any individual with hypertrichosis or hirsutism should be thoroughly investigated for potential hormonal imbalances, familial hypertrichosis or medication use. The individual's skin type and hair color help predict the response to treatment and determine which laser device is more suitable for each patient.[10] The best results are achieved with light-skinned, dark-haired individuals. For patients with darker skin complexion, pretreatment with a bleaching cream or tretinoin may make the treatment safer and more effective. In sun-tanned individuals, treatment should be deferred, as any amount of suntan increases the risk of adverse effects, such as blisters or scarring. The procedure is well tolerated and does not usually require anesthesia, although topical anesthetics can be used in the treatment of large surface areas or sensitive regions, for example upper lip, bikini area. Patients should be informed that multiple treatments are required in order to obtain complete hair removal, and that the exact number of treatments varies among different anatomic sites.[11]

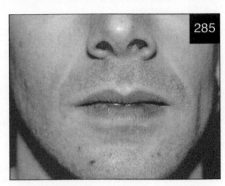

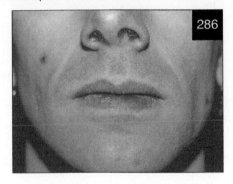

285: Prior to laser hair removal.
286: After six laser hair removal sessions with long-pulsed ruby laser of the entire face except for the moustache area.

Side effects and complications

Laser hair removal is a relatively safe procedure. Complications are rare, provided that patients are carefully selected, appropriate guidelines have been followed, and the treatment performed by physicians or supervised medical staff. Pain, erythema, and swelling occur in virtually all patients after laser treatment and usually resolve after 1–3 days. Blistering and crusting are rare and may lead to postinflammatory changes, particularly in patients with darker skin phototype (IV–V) or with a suntan. Reactivation of labial herpes infection, blistering and crusting may also occur. Scarring has not been reported but remains a possible adverse event if high fluences are used or postoperative infections occur. All patients should avoid direct sun exposure after treatment and should use a high SPF sunscreen.

References

1. Zensie HH, Altshuler GB, Smirnov MZ, Anderson RR. Evaluation of cooling methods for laser dermatology. *Lasers Surg Med* 2000;**26**:130–44.

2. Eremia S, Li CY, Umar SH, Newman N. Laser hair removal: long-term results with a 755 nm alexandrite laser. *Dermatol Surg* 2001;**27**:920–4.

3. Fiskerstrand EJ, Svaasand LO, Nelson JS. Hair removal with long pulsed diode lasers: a comparison between two systems with different pulse structures. *Lasers Surg Med* 2003;**32**:399-404.

4. Tanzi EL, Alster TS. Long-pulsed 1064-nm Nd:YAG laser-assisted hair removal in all skin types. *Dermatol Surg* 2004;**30**:13-17.

5. Sadick NS, Weiss RA, Shea CR, Nagel H, Nicholson J, Prieto VG. Long-term photoepilation using a broad spectrum intense pulsed light source. *Arch Dermatol* 2000;**136**.1336–40.

6. Dierickx CC, Grossman MC, Farinelli WA *et* al. Permanent hair removal by normal-mode ruby laser. *Arch Dermatol* 1998;**134**:837–44.

7. Handrick C, Alster TS. Comparison of long-pulsed diode and long-pulsed alexandrite lasers for hair removal: a long-term clinical and histological study. *Dermatol Surg* 2001;**27**:622-626.

8. Grossman MC, Lou WW, Geronemus RG et al. Long term comparison of different lasers and light sources for hair removal. *Lasers Surg Med* 2000;**12**(Suppl.):89.

9. Ross EV, Cooke LM, Timko AL, Overstreet KA, Graham BS, Barnette DJ. Treatment of pseudofolliculitis barbae in skin types IV, V, and VI with a long-pulsed neodymium:yttrium aluminum garnet laser. J Am *Acad Dermatol* 2002;**47**:263-270.

10. Liew SH. Laser hair removal: guidelines for management. Am J *Clin Dermatol* 2002;**3**:107-115.

11. Dierickx CC. Hair removal by lasers and intense pulsed light sources. *Dermatol Clin* 2001;**20**:135–6.

Table 25.1: **Laser or light source selection for hair removal**

Hair color	Skin type	Laser/light source
Dark-colored (fine)	Fair	Ruby (694 nm) Alexandrite (755 nm) Intense pulsed light source
Dark-colored (coarse)	Fair	Diode (810 nm) Long pulse Nd:YAG (1064 nm) Ruby (694 nm) Alexandrite (755 nm) Intense pulsed light source
Dark-colored	Dark	Diode (810 nm) Long pulse Nd:YAG (1064 nm) Intense pulsed light source
Red, blond or gray	Fair	All commercially available laser devices produce temporary hair loss
White	Fair/dark	Carbon-Q switched Nd:YAG laser (temporary hair loss) Photodynamic therapy

Index

Printed and bound by CPI Group (UK) Ltd, Croydon, CR0 4YY

23/10/2024

01777682-0013